SURVIVING CANCER

A HOLISTIC APPROACH TO FOCUSING ON YOUR BODY AND MIND FOR TOTAL HEALING

ALLYSON WARK MD PhD

INTRODUCTION

The course of events can occasionally be determined by the biology of a tumor rather than the patient's outlook or spirit of resistance. Often, we have no influence over these occurrences. However, individuals who have a positive outlook are better able to manage the symptoms of their diseases and may benefit more from therapy. Many doctors have witnessed the striking differences in outcomes between two patients with comparable diagnoses, degrees of disease, and treatment regimens. The fact that one patient is pessimistic and the other optimistic is one of the few obvious contrasts.

There is a clear connection between the mind, the body, and one's health, as has been understood for more than 2,000 years thanks to Plato and Galen's writings. Plato concluded, "Doctors are uninformed of the remedy for many ailments because they are ignorant of the entire, Since the component cannot be healthy until the entire is"

The recognition of this wisdom—that the psychological and physical components of the body are interdependent parts of a whole system rather than being distinct, unrelated, and separate—has recently occurred in the field of health care. Health is increasingly understood to be a result of a complex interaction between a variety of factors, including genetics, environment, emotional and psychological states, dietary patterns, and exercise routines.

Chapter 1

Overview of cancer

The term "cancer" is broad. It explains the illness that develops as a result of unchecked cell growth and division brought on by cellular alterations. While certain cancer types cause cells to grow and divide more slowly than others, some cancer types promote fast cell growth. While certain cancers, like leukemia, may not cause visible growths known as tumors, others, like carcinoma, do. The majority of cells in the body have specific purposes and lifespans. Although it may seem harmful, cell death is a normal and advantageous process known as apoptosis. A cell is given the go-ahead to pass away so that the body can swap it out for a younger, more functional cell. Cancerous cells are lacking in the elements that tell healthy cells to stop growing and to die. As a result, they gather throughout the body and feed on nutrients and oxygen that would ordinarily feed other cells. Tumors, immune system impairment, and other changes brought on by cancerous cells can prevent the body from operating normally. The lymph nodes may allow cancerous cells to spread from where they first appeared. Immune cell colonies can be seen all over the body. The onset of cancer may be influenced by genetic factors.

The genetic coding in a person determines when their cells will divide and die. Gene changes may result in incorrect instructions, which may cause cancer. Proteins carry many of the instructions for cellular growth and division, and genes can also affect how proteins are produced by the cells. Certain genes alter the proteins that would typically mend harmed cells. This might result in cancer. The changed instructions could be passed on to a child if a parent carries these genes. Some genetic alterations take place after birth, and risks might be increased by things like smoking and sun exposure. The chemical signals that control how the body uses, or "expresses," particular genes undergo other alterations that can result in cancer. Finally, a propensity to a certain type of cancer might be inherited. This can be referred to as having a hereditary cancer syndrome by a doctor. The 5–10 most prevalent types of cancer cases are heavily influenced by inherited genetic alterations, according to a reliable source.

According to the National Cancer Institute, which excluded non melanoma skin cancer from these findings, breast cancer is the most prevalent type of cancer in the U.S., followed by lung and prostate cancer.

One of the following cancers is diagnosed in more than 40,000 persons nationwide each year:

• Bladder

• Gastro Intestinal tract

• Endometrial

• Kidney

• Leukemia

• Liver

• Melanoma

• Non-Hodgkin lymphoma

• Pancreatic

• Thyroid

Less frequent are other kinds. The National Cancer Institute estimates that there are over 100 reliable origins of cancer.

Signs and Symptoms of Cancer

Cancer symptoms and warning signals might include:

- Fever

- Pain

- Fatigue

- Skin alterations (redness, un-healing wounds, jaundice, darkening)

- Unintentional weight gain or reduction

Other, more blatant indications of cancer might include:

- Tumors or lumps (mass)

- Trouble swallowing

- Modifications to or issues with bowel or bladder function

- Chronic coughing or hoarseness

- Breathing difficulty

- Chest ache

- Unaccounted for hemorrhage or discharge

Cell division and cancer development

Cancer is categorized according to;

• It's location in the body.

• The tissues in which it develops

Sarcomas, for instance, arise in bones or soft tissues, whereas carcinomas do so in the cells that covers the body's internal or external surfaces. Adenocarcinomas can grow in the breast, whereas basal cell carcinomas can develop in the skin.

Metastasis is the medical word for the process by which malignant cells spread to different regions of the body.

Additionally, a person may be battling many cancers at once.

The intricate process through which cancerous cells arise from healthy cells is known as malignant transformation. These are the steps in it:

• Initiation

• Promotion

• Spread

Initiation

Initiation is the first stage of cancer growth, during which a mutation in a cell's genetic make-up prepares it to produce cancer. The genetic material of the cell may alter spontaneously or as a result of a cancer-causing substance (a carcinogen). Numerous chemicals, cigarettes, viruses, radiation, and sunlight are all carcinogens. Not all cells, though, are equally vulnerable to carcinogens. A cell may be more vulnerable if it has a genetic defect that was either inherited or acquired. Even mild physical irritability over time can increase a cell's susceptibility to carcinogens.

Promotion

Promotion is the second and last stage in the growth of cancer. Environmental elements or even some drugs, like sex hormones, can act as promoters or agents that produce promotion (for example, testosterone taken to improve sex drive and energy in older men). Promoters do not by themselves cause cancer, unlike carcinogens. Instead, promoters permit a malignant cell to spread after it has experienced initiation. Cells that have not undergone initiation are unaffected by promotion. Some carcinogens are potent enough to cause cancer without needing to be promoted. In particular, sarcomas, leukemia, thyroid cancer, and breast cancer can all be brought on by ionizing radiation, which is used in x-rays and produced in nuclear power plants and atomic bomb blasts.

Spread

Cancer can spread to nearby or distant tissues or organs or grow into (invade) surrounding tissue directly. The lymphatic system can help cancer spread. Carcinomas commonly spread in this manner. For instance, breast cancer typically spreads first to the local armpit lymph nodes before moving on to distant places. Bloodstream circulation can also help cancer spread. Sarcomas frequently spread in this manner.

Stages of cancer

One of the following five stages often corresponds to the TNM categorization of a malignancy.

•Stage 0: This describes cancer that is "in situ," or constrained to the area where it first developed. This particular malignancy has not invaded more tissues or spread.

• Stages I through III: These advanced stages of cancer are characterized by bigger tumors and/or a more severe course of the illness. When cancer is in this stage, it may have already invaded nearby lymph nodes, tissues, or organs.

•Stage IV: This stage of cancer refers to the spread of the disease to distant lymph nodes, bodily tissues, or organs.

CYCLE OF CANCER CELLS

Compared to healthy cells in the body, cancer cells behave differently. Numerous of these variations are influenced by how cells divide. For instance, cancer cells can proliferate in culture (outside the body in a plate) without the addition of growth factors or protein signals that stimulate growth. This is in opposition to normal cells, which require growth hormones in order to replicate in vitro. Cancer cells may produce their own growth factors; have growth factor pathways that are permanently turned on, or, depending on the body's environment, may even fool nearby cells into making growth factors so they may survive. Additionally, cancer cells don't stop replicating and thus disobey signals in the body telling them to stop. For instance, normal cells cultured in a plate that are surrounded by neighbors cease to divide. In contrast, cancer cells continue to divide and form lumpy layers on top of one another. Though the conditions in a dish and the human body are very different, researchers believe that the absence of contact inhibition in plate-grown cancer cells is a reflection of the absence of a process that normally keeps tissue balance in the body. The "replicative immortality," a fancy word meaning the ability to divide significantly more than a normal bodily cell, is another characteristic of cancer cells. Human cells may typically divide only 40–60 times before they lose the ability to do so, "age," and ultimately perish. Cancer cells are able to divide far more frequently than usual, in large part because they produce the enzyme telomerase, which prevents the normal wearing down of chromosomal ends during cell division. In addition, cancer cells differ from healthy cells in several indirect ways unrelated to the cell cycle. They multiply, divide, and develop tumors thanks to these variations. For instance, cancer cells acquire the capacity to spread throughout the body (a process known as metastasis) and to encourage the development of new blood vessels (a process known as angiogenesis) (which gives tumor cells a source of oxygen and nutrients). Additionally, cancer cells resist going through apoptosis, or programmed cell death, when normal cells would (e.g., due to DNA damage). Additionally, recent studies have revealed that cancer cells may experience metabolic alterations that promote faster cell growth and division. Additionally, cancer cells disobey signals that should make them stop proliferating. For instance, normal cells cultured in a plate that are surrounded by neighbors cease to divide. In contrast, cancer cells continue to divide and form lumpy layers on top of one another. Cells have a variety of methods that they can use to control cell division, fix DNA damage, and stop the growth of cancer. As a result, it is believed that the development of cancer occurs through a number of steps and requires the failure of several different mechanisms before a critical mass of malignant cells is reached. To be more precise, the majority of cancers develop when cells experience a succession of mutations (changes in DNA) that cause them to reproduce more rapidly, circumvent internal and external restrictions on division, and resist programmed cell death.

In a fictitious scenario, a cell might first lose the ability to halt the cell cycle, which would cause the cell's offspring to divide a little more quickly. Although it is doubtful that they would be cancerous, they could develop a benign tumor, which is a collection of cells that divide excessively but are not able to spread to other tissues (metastasize). One of the descendent cells may experience a mutation throughout time, increasing the activity of a positive cell cycle regulator. Even though the mutation might not be cancer-causing on its own, the children of this cell would divide even more quickly, expanding the population of cells in which a third mutation might occur. One cell may eventually develop enough mutations to resemble a cancer cell and develop into a malignant tumor, a collection of cells that divide rapidly and have the ability to infiltrate other tissues. Typically, a tumor's cells develop more mutations as it grows. Large-scale mutations like the duplication or deletion of entire chromosomes are examples of large-scale mutations that may occur in the genomes of malignancies that are in an advanced stage. How do these alterations occur? They appear to be caused, at least in some instances, by inactivating mutations in the very genes that maintain the stability of the genome (that is, genes that stop mutations from happening or being passed on). These genes produce proteins that perform a variety of essential maintenance functions, including detecting and repairing DNA damage, blocking substances that attach to DNA, protecting chromosomal ends called telomeres, and more. These genes can develop several mutations very quickly if one of them is damaged and dysfunctional. Therefore, offspring of a cell with a dysfunctional genome stability factor may accumulate the necessary number of mutations for cancer much more quickly than do normal cells.

Cancer and cell cycle regulators

Each every tumor has a distinct set of genetic abnormalities, and many cancer forms entail various sorts of mutations. Negative regulators, also known as tumor suppressors, may be inactivated while positive regulators, also known as oncogenic regulators, may be over activated (become oncogenic).

Oncogenes

In cancer, positive cell cycle regulators might be hyperactive. For instance, a cyclin may express at abnormally high levels, or a growth factor receptor may send signals even when no growth factors are present. Oncogenes are the hyperactive (cancer-promoting) variants of these genes, whereas proto-oncogenes are the normal, un-mutated forms. This nomenclature reflects the fact that an oncogene can develop from a normal proto-oncogene if it undergoes a mutation that boosts its activity. Different types of mutations can transform proto-oncogenes into oncogenes. Some modify the protein's amino acid sequence, changing its structure and keeping it in a "always on" state. Others involve amplification, where a cell acquires extra copies of a gene and then begins to produce an excessive amount of protein. In yet other situations, a mistake in DNA repair may join a proto-oncogene to a section of another gene, resulting in a "combo" protein with uncontrolled activity.

Proto-oncogenes are responsible for encoding a large number of the proteins that carry growth factor signals. These proteins typically only promote cell cycle progression in the presence of growth factors. However, if one of the proteins develops a hyperactive state as a result of a mutation, it might still send signals even if there are no growth factors present. Proto-oncogenes all encode the growth factor receptor, Ras protein, and signaling enzyme Raf. These proteins frequently take on overactive versions in cancer cells. For instance, roughly 90% of pancreatic tumors have oncogenic Ras mutations. Ras is a G protein, which means that it alternates between an active and inactive state while coupled to the tiny molecule GDP (bound to the similar molecule GTP). Ras's structure is frequently altered by cancer-causing mutations, making it incapable of switching to its inactive form or able to do so only extremely slowly, keeping the protein in an active state.

Suppressors of tumors

In cancer cells, negative cell cycle regulators may be less active or even inactive. For instance, a protein that normally senses DNA damage and stops the advancement of the cell cycle may no longer do so. Tumor suppressor genes are those that ordinarily prevent the advancement of the cell cycle. When tumor suppressors function properly, they prevent the growth of malignant tumors, whereas cancers can develop when they mutate and cease to function. Tumor protein p53, one of the most significant tumor suppressors, is crucial to the cellular response to DNA damage. In reaction to DNA damage and other adverse circumstances, p53 slows cell cycle progression at the G_1 checkpoint (regulating the G_1 to S transition). A sensor protein that detects DNA damage activates p53, which causes the creation of a cell-cycle inhibitor to commence at the G_1 checkpoint and stop the cell cycle. This interlude gives DNA repair, which is also dependent on p53, which also functions as a DNA repair enzyme activator, some breathing room. If the harm is repaired, p53 will let go, allowing the cell to proceed through the cell cycle. If the damage cannot be repaired, p53 will perform its third and final function, which is to cause apoptosis (planned cell death), preventing the transmission of damaged DNA. Normal p53 attaches to DNA and encourages transcription of target genes in response to DNA damage. In order to give time for repairs, p53 first causes the creation of Cdk inhibitor proteins, which causes the cell cycle to pause in G1. Additionally, p53 stimulates DNA repair mechanisms. Finally, p53 initiates apoptosis if DNA repair is not feasible. The overall result of p53's actions is to prevent the inheritance of damaged DNA, either by causing the cell to self-destruct or by getting the damage repaired. When a cell simply has defective p53, which is unable to bind DNA, none of these three reactions are still triggered by DNA damage. Even though the damage still activates p53, it is powerless to react since it can no longer control the transcription of its targets. As a result, apoptosis is not triggered, DNA damage is not repaired, and the cell does not pause in G1. Overall, the absence of p53 causes damaged DNA (mutations) to be transmitted to daughter cells. P53 is frequently absent, dysfunctional, or less active than usual in cancer cells. For instance, the p53 gene has been altered so that it can no longer bind DNA in many malignant tumors. The non-binding mutant protein cannot function because p53 regulates transcription by binding to target genes. A cell with damaged DNA may continue to divide when p53 is malfunctioning. Due to the mother cell's unrepaired DNA, the daughter cells of such a division are likely to inherit mutations. Cells with defective p53 have a propensity to develop mutations across generations, some of which can transform proto-oncogenes into oncogenes or deactivate other tumor suppressors. Human tumors most frequently include mutations in the p53 gene, while cancer cells without these mutations most likely inactivate p53 by different mechanisms (e.g., increased activity of the proteins that cause p53 to be recycled).

Chapter 2

Breaking the news

It can be overwhelming to learn that you have cancer, both for you and for your friends and family. People frequently lack the words to say. They might be depressed, uneasy, and scared of upsetting you. They might be concerned that they might lose you. Because they are worried about saying the wrong thing, some people find it easier to remain silent. Speaking comes naturally to some people, whereas others might become overly cautious or act too cheerful. As you learn more about your diagnosis and start learning about treatment options, you'll probably experience a wide range of emotions. It's normal to feel sad, angry, or afraid, or to wonder, "Why me?" Your feelings can also be influenced by physical and chemical changes brought on by chemotherapy or the cancer itself. Admitting your feelings to yourself is the first step, and allowing yourself to feel how you do is acceptable.

Preparing to converse with others.

You alone will determine when to inform your loved ones that you are suffering from cancer. The news that someone has cancer will definitely shock everyone.

When in a situation like this, most people need and want to talk to someone. In the case of a single person without supportive family members, telling close friends what is going on will even be more crucial. When someone asks how they can help, prepare an answer in advance because people who live alone frequently have a few more demands than those who live with others. Informing your loved ones might occasionally help you come to terms with the reality of what is happening. Some people discover that as their family and friends ask questions, they start to think about other issues and start to solve problems. Consider how much you want to divulge. You might want to describe the type of cancer you have, any potential treatments, and your prognosis (or prognosis). Write down any questions you have as you converse with others so you can discuss them with your cancer care team later.

Selecting a recipient

Making a list of the people you want to speak with in person may be a good place to start. Then you can make another list of friends who you see less frequently and tell another friend or member of your family to get in touch with them. Before telling other family members and close friends, people typically tell their spouse or partner. Additionally, it's crucial to inform your kids, which may take additional planning depending on their age. If you work, consider how much information your coworkers need to know and whether you want to share it with them. Although you may need to inform a supervisor or a member of human resources that you have a medical issue if you need time off, coworkers and friends frequently learn about it afterwards. Different people need knowledge at different levels. If you do choose to notify your coworkers, you might start by speaking with and seeking advice from a trusted colleague. Some people inform their group of coworkers at a meeting or via a carefully crafted email so that everyone has a basic knowledge of what is going on. There isn't a single correct response that applies to everyone; it all depends on your preferences and the working culture.

Discussing cancer with others

Tell your loved ones how you're feeling in general. It can be challenging, but it's beneficial to let others know when you're unhappy, anxious, angry, or experiencing other emotional problems. You might want to look for a support group or a mental health professional to assist you if you don't feel comfortable doing this. Your support group or counselor will be available for you at a regular time set out for you to concentrate on and discuss your challenges. Others favor peer support networks, workshops, or religious guidance.

Look for what works for you.

You should undergo self-awareness and until you find out what works for you, but till then try out various things .It lessens your load when you keep others informed about your disease and involved. It can be beneficial for everyone concerned if friends and family can express their support and concern for you and for one another. Please keep in mind that it's perfectly acceptable to hold back on certain topics if you or your family isn't typically comfortable discussing them. Some people use extreme caution while choosing their conversation partners and topics. But this could be a good time for you to work on opening up to trusted family members.

Giving specifics

It could get tiresome to repeatedly explain your ailment to a large number of individuals. As an alternative to spending hours on the phone updating friends and family, there are websites specifically created for cancer patients and their families, such as "CaringBridge." These websites often provide you the option to control who may view your updates; you can either make them public or restrict access to those you specifically invite. Ask a family member or trusted friend who is familiar with these websites and tools for assistance if you are unable to set it up yourself. To inform friends of updates or changes, some people send group emails, texts, or tweets. Some websites even offer to send emails or texts on your behalf. This can reduce the number of calls made while still providing information to those who care or are simply inquisitive.

Find out what "triggers" you.

Consider your "trigger points," or subjects that are still too delicate for you to discuss. Do you become irate when people criticize your medical decisions? Maybe this should be a subject you'll have to avoid. Does it annoy you when people bring religion into it, saying things like, "God never gives you more than you can handle?" Think about the things that people have said or could say that bother you. Plan a response that will cut off the conversation and be comfortable for you. And once you've said what you wanted to say, be ready to switch to a different subject. You could say, "I really get uncomfortable of talking about cancer." Let's discuss something different.

Inquire about their opinions.

Encourage family members to share their feelings with you so you can discuss them and find solutions. How are you? Can be also be used as a greeting. Do you really believe this? This enables your friend or relative to discuss their emotions with you. However, don't ask if you're not ready to learn about their worries and fears. Managing your treatment and determining how you feel can be difficult enough without having to consider other people. It requires work—effort and emotional work— that you might not be able to put forth. But this is one way to encourage openness if you want to. You might not always want to discuss how you feel or how others are feeling. Simply stating, "You know, usually I am OK talking about things like this, but today I just can't handle it," will be sufficient to politely convey this to others. You must understand, and I'm sure that by doing this, you can decide for yourself when and under what conditions you can talk about your illness.

When others desire to assist

What can I do to help? Is frequently one of the first questions asked by friend or family member. There is the temptation to respond, "Oh, nothing at the moment I'm perfectly fine". It's possible that you don't really know what you need, that you desire your privacy, or that you believe you have enough going on without more people in your life. Keep in mind that most people genuinely want to assist you, and that during your cancer treatment, you may undoubtedly require additional assistance at some point. Be as specific as you can about the type of assistance you require. Inquire if they can assist with housecleaning, yard work, or child care, for instance, or let them know when you need a ride to the doctor. Even just expressing that you don't know what you need will be helpful at times. They have an opportunity to offer something they can do for you as well.

When others make hurtful remarks and tell you to be happy.

When you chat to your friends or family about your unhappiness, concerns, or anxieties, they could encourage you to "cheer up." It's acceptable to politely inquire whether they would be willing to simply listen without passing judgment or offering advice (unless you ask for it). It's important for your mental health that you find someone you can talk to. Do not let those who are uncomfortable with your feelings demotivate you. Some people can't listen because of their own experiences or their own pain, not because of you. You are not involved in any of that. You might have to concede that this individual isn't the greatest one to talk to about some things. Seek out those who are better able to handle it.

Pose inquiries you don't want to respond to.

When you don't feel like answering questions about your cancer, you might discover that occasionally you have to. You might want to ask a relative or friend to serve as your spokesperson in order to prevent this. Repeating your sickness to everyone who is worried about you can be emotionally draining. Having a spokesman spares you from doing this and keeps family members informed without draining you of energy. Your cancer diagnosis could occasionally make "huge news" in your neighborhood. People are frequently genuinely concerned even though they don't know you well. Naturally, there are those who are merely curious. Cancer is a highly private illness, so you should feel comfortable sharing only as much as is necessary with others who merely want to be informed. You might need to consider how to politely inform others that you don't want to discuss matters that are private. Many times, simply saying "Thank you for asking, but I'd rather not talk about it right now" will be sufficient to get your point across, but occasionally you may need to be more forthright. It can be necessary to say, "I'd prefer not to go into details" or "I don't want to delve into my private health difficulties." Consider how you wish to respond to enquiring remarks from strangers. Consider coming up with a response that suits you.

Unexpectedly bring up of cancer

People will occasionally make an effort to make you feel better on days when you are really upset. Another possibility is that while you're trying to concentrate on your child's school play, someone approaches you and begins talking about their disease. Perhaps a stranger you hardly know approaches you in the grocery store and breaks the awful news of her father's sickness. Even when you truly don't want to hear their story, you know they're just being polite or trying to connect with you. How can you respectfully stop them? Sometimes you just need to gently respond, "Thank you very much for your care, but I need to focus on something else today," after taking a few deep breaths. Never forget that the decision to discuss something is always your own.

Loved ones becoming irritated or frustrated with you

Sometimes, folks who are close to you can also get furious. Others nearby might be experiencing similar sentiments to you, just as you are experiencing a wide range of emotions. The majority of people may experience anger at some point, but try to remember that your loved ones are furious with the circumstance, not with you. Most likely, you experience the same thing occasionally. "You are not doing the things you used to do," someone may say. Some kids and even some adults can be very egotistical. As you start to concentrate on treatment and healing, your social, family, and professional roles will shift. You might not be able to do what you have been doing at times because of low energy levels. If you explain this to the individuals around you and discuss your feelings about the various changes occurring in your life, you will adjust more readily. Tell your family that even though you won't be able to complete all of the tasks alone, they can still be completed.

Maintain as much normalcy as you can.

Allow yourself and your family members to maintain as much normalcy as you can while you are receiving therapy. Encourage your family to continue living the way they have without feeling bad (enjoying hobbies, playing sports, exercising, spending time with friends, and so on). The practice is especially beneficial for kids, but it also gives adults grounding for day-to-day living.

What to avoid:

•Don't shun or neglect a friend or family member who might need to confide in you.

•Pay attention to your personal need for human contact.

•If you don't truly feel that way, don't put on a "happy face" or a false front. Even though you might have a tendency to put on a happy front to try to shield your loved ones, sharing your actual emotions will benefit both you and them.

• believe there is a right or wrong way to conduct yourself in social situations. You'll notice that there are moments when talking and sharing make you feel terrific and other times when that feeling is not as strong. Recognize that, for the most part, you and others are doing the best you can. And that's sufficient.

When to consult a physician

Your therapy may occasionally cause physical side effects, and if this happens, your cancer care team may be able to assist you. Learn more about the physical side effects and symptoms of cancer therapy, as well as when you should seek assistance. Cancer and the stress it causes might start to make some people feel as though life isn't worth living. If you have any thoughts of injuring yourself, please speak with your doctor or nurse as soon as possible. Many patients require additional assistance and support to get through cancer and cancer treatments, which can be difficult.

Chapter 3

Psychosocial and emotional approach to cancer

There are a number of reasons why a cancer patient could choose not to seek treatment for their mental health condition: It might be challenging to distinguish between cancer, depression, and anxiety because they overlap symptoms including exhaustion, lack of sleep, and decreased appetite. It can be challenging to distinguish between indicators of a mental health disorder and normal reactions to a cancer diagnosis and treatment in this group of people who frequently confront threats to their lives. Teams who treat cancer patients frequently lack the expertise to identify mental health issues. There is disagreement in the community on what depression is and looks like. Many people are compelled to view their mental health as less essential and do not seek help since cancer treatment takes so much time and money.

Cancer can have an impact on your mind as well as your physical health, and many people will notice substantial changes in their emotional well-being. A person's and their loved ones' reactions to learning they have cancer can be profound, and depressive, anxious, and fearful emotions are frequently experienced. But it's crucial to keep in mind that there are hope, support, and treatment options for many types of mental illness. It does not make a person's depression any less treatable just because they may also have cancer. Everyone is aware that early detection of cancer at stage one is preferable to late detection at stage four. The same is true for illnesses related to mental health. Unfortunately, many cancer patients are never informed of the possibility that they might have a mental health problem like depression and are not given therapy for it.

Cancer patients frequently experience not just physical and mental suffering as a result of their diagnosis and treatment, but also significant changes to their everyday routines. As a result, patients frequently experience issues with numerous facets of social life, including relationships with family, friends, coworkers, employers, income, leisure activities, and healthcare professionals. The length of hospital stays for cancer patients has decreased as a result of recent advancements in medical technology and the accessibility of outpatient care. The primary location of cancer patient treatment is anticipated to shift more and more from hospitals to homes in the future as terminal home care is anticipated to be more widely encouraged. Under these conditions, cancer patients and their families must deal with a variety of social issues that develop as the disease and treatment advance. Social wellbeing may be adversely threatened by cancer and its treatment. Data from several research studies were combined to indicate that 45 percent of cancer patients experienced high levels of social difficulty, including issues with social interactions and support, loneliness, limitations on social activities, difficulties at work, and obligations outside of work. Managing at home, health and welfare services, finances, jobs, legal issues, relationships, sexuality and body image, and recreation are some of the social issues that cancer patients deal with. Cancer has an impact on patients' social relationships, including those with their spouses, friends, and family. Patients' social connections, which frequently serve as unofficial caregivers, can support patients as they deal with the effects of their sickness. Although providing informal care is a worthwhile endeavor, it may also be taxing. Social repercussions from informal caregivers' caregiving practices are common. Additionally, they encounter resistance from their social connections and find it difficult to discuss the malignancy with others. Additionally, it appears that informal caregivers engage in fewer social activities because they feel guilty or anxious when they are apart from the patient. According to a recent analysis, informal caregivers also benefit socially by caring for someone who has cancer, such as improving their bond with the patient.

A cancer diagnosis is a life-changing event, and cancer patients go through physical as well as psychological changes. Patients with cancer frequently experience anxiety, sleeplessness, exhaustion, and despair, as well as general mental anguish, which can result in social issues with intimacy, communicating with others, or body image. PTSD is increasingly being identified in cancer patients as well. For instance, dealing with a procedure like a mastectomy or limb amputation can result in PTSD in a cancer patient. A lengthy chemotherapy regimen with side effects including hair loss or neuropathy can also cause psychological discomfort in patients (nerve pain or numbness). PTSD is more likely to occur in cancer patients who have required prolonged critical care unit stays. Examples include a young breast cancer patient who experiences fatigue and depressive symptoms during chemotherapy or an elderly patient who is overwhelmed by managing the demands of living with an ostomy after surgery to treat bladder cancer. It's crucial in helping cancer patients cope with the demands and stresses of both an initial cancer diagnosis and managing behavioral complications associated with cancer treatments. Patients must be aware of the psychological impacts that the disease will have on them as well as how to combat those effects throughout the frequently lengthy cancer treatment, which may involve numerous different therapies such as surgery, chemotherapy, radiation therapy, and immunotherapy. To ensure that psychosocial oncology therapy is ongoing, self-care should extend from initial treatments and into remission and finally survivorship. Therapy of all kinds, such as supportive psychotherapy, cognitive behavioral psychotherapy, and interpersonal therapy, might be beneficial. Major depression is treated using these three different psychotherapies on cancer patients, both men and women, and it has been found that all three methods work well. Hospitalized patients with acute psychiatric problems such delirium, sometimes known as an acute confused state, depression, and anxiety can be treated. Palliative care and pain management are essential to address pain, anxiety, and co-occurring mental disorders in patients with complex pain syndromes since they are frequently very distressed. Working closely with their outpatient mental health providers will help cancer patients with severe and persistent mental illnesses, such as schizophrenia; manage their psychosocial and psychiatric care within the context of their cancer treatment. Despite the fact that most survivors manage their lives effectively, individuals occasionally experience psychosocial disorders that might manifest as symptoms like persistent weariness, a loss of attention or stamina, or sexual dysfunction. Psychological themes in cancer survivors may include a persistent feeling of vulnerability and uncertainty about a potential recurrence. It is crucial that cancer survivors have regular psychosocial assessments and psychosocial care as needed. Online platforms and other group support interventions are frequently helpful to survivors. Occasionally, survivors may exhibit depressive symptoms that, after a thorough evaluation, result in a new medical diagnosis that explains the symptoms, such as depression or anxiety. In other words, the goal of psychosocial oncology is to make sure that patients receive ongoing attention for coping, distress, and quality of life, including all medical and psycho-social aspects of cancer survivorship.

Psychological disorders and management techniques for each.

Depression

Depression affects patient outcomes and lowers quality of life, and also raises the death risk for cancer patients. It's estimated that cancer patients experience depression at a rate up to three times higher than the general population. It has been discovered that depressed individuals may experience worse cancer-related outcomes. They can be less inclined to adhere to treatment schedules or go through screenings. For instance, they might miss therapy visits, exercise less, or consume too much alcohol. According to studies, those who have dementia, severe mental illness, or substance abuse are more likely to have a decreased likelihood of surviving after receiving a cancer diagnosis. There is excellent reason to assume that mental health treatment may be able to alter the course of cancer, which is a question that many specialists are asking. According to one study, people who received treatment and had fewer depressive symptoms lived longer on average than people with more symptoms. People who receive therapy frequently see improvements in their overall health, are more likely to continue receiving care, and have a higher quality of life. To improve quality of life and lower mortality, there is a critical need to recognize and treat depression in cancer patients. We briefly cover the most prominent clinical and prospective future biochemical screening methods for cancer depression. The interventions utilized will differ for each patient, but may include pharmacological or psychosocial therapies. The best mix of therapies is uncertain due to a lack of research on the most effective management of depression in cancer patients.

Symptoms of depression.

For at least two weeks, the patient must exhibit either a sad mood or a diminished degree of interest or enjoyment in activities. Additionally, four or more of the following requirements must be met:

•Substantial weight loss,

•Alterations in the mind-body,

•Fatigue,

•Negative self-esteem,

•Poor mental capacity

•Recurring ideas of suicide or death.

- Anxious or depressed mood

- Sleep issues (i.e., sleeping too much or too little; sleeping mainly during the day)

- A shift in interests (i.e., losing interest in things you once like) or a lack of motivation

- Excessive guilt or an unreasonably low opinion of oneself

- Noticeably decreased energy or a shift in self-care (i.e., not showering anymore)

- Significantly reduced focus (i.e., sharp decline in performance)

- Alterations in appetite (i.e., eating too much or too little)

- Excessive agitation or panic attacks

- Suicidal ideas, and self-harm (i.e., intentionally cutting or hurting yourself)

It's critical to keep in mind that not all people who are depressed attempt suicide. Even if you haven't shown any specific signs of self-harm or suicide conducts, or if your symptoms aren't as severe or chronic as those mentioned above, you can still get help. Additionally, the symptoms must be severe enough to cause significant distress or impairment and not be brought on by a disease or its physiological side effects. Clinical professionals may mistake the bodily signs of depression, such as exhaustion, lack of appetite, weight shift, and impaired cognition, for side effects of cancer therapy or other illnesses, which results in a reduction in the disorder's identification. One study indicated that, even after controlling for cancer pain and physical functionality, changes in appetite and decreased cognitive performance were positively associated with anhedonia, whereas sleep problems and weariness were not. This shows that decreased appetite and poor cognition might be better indicators of depression in cancer patients. Sad cancer patients have lower levels of shame and failure feelings (4%) compared to depressed patients who are otherwise healthy (56.5%). Given the severe physical and psychological stress on patients, it may be normal for some of the symptoms listed above to be present, making diagnosis difficult. Other behavioral issues that patients may struggle with include exhaustion, poor cognition, anorexia, social disengagement, and sleep problems.

Controlling depression

Counseling, medicine, or a combination of the two, along with occasionally other specialist treatments, may be used to address depression in cancer patients. These therapies alleviate the cancer patient's depression, ease their pain, and enhance their quality of life.

• Discuss your emotions and any worries you or your family members may have. Feeling depressed, irate, or frustrated is acceptable, but try not to vent your emotions on those who are important to you. It's critical to pay close attention to one another's words, come to a consensus on how you might support one another, and encourage rather than coerce one another to speak.

• Look for assistance through counseling and support organizations.

• Use spiritual practices such as prayer, meditation, or mindfulness.

• Several times per day, practice deep breathing and relaxation techniques. (For instance, close your eyes, take a deep breath, and then concentrate on and relax each part of your body, starting with your toes and working your way up to your head. Imagine yourself at a lovely location when you're at ease, like a sunny meadow or a breezy beach.

• If you want help adjusting to the changes in your life, think about talking with a professional counselor.

• Depression treatments and drugs should only be used when prescribed by a medical professional and should not conflict with chemotherapy.

How family members can assist

• Invite the patient to speak kindly about their worries and fears. Never compel a patient to speak before they are ready.

• Listen intently without passing judgment on the patient's or your own emotions. It's acceptable to call attention to and reject negative beliefs.

• Refrain from encouraging them to "cheer up" or "think optimistically."

• Agree on what you can each do to support the other.

• If the person is experiencing significant dread, anxiety, or sadness, don't try to reason with them. Consult a member of the cancer care team for assistance.

• Participate in activities that individual enjoys.

• Bear in mind that caregivers can experience depression as well. All of these recommendations are also applicable to carers.

• Schedule some time for self-care. Engage in activities you enjoy or spend time with friends.

• Take into account seeking out group or one-on-one counseling as a form of self-support.

If the patient has cancer, and is having any of these signs below contact the cancer care team or the mental health practitioner.

• Has suicidal ideas or is always thinking about death

• Acts in a way that makes you worry about their safety.

• For several days, they are unable to eat or sleep or show any interest in their typical activities.

• Has difficulty breathing, is perspiring, or appears to be very restless

Getting Over Depression

Use these coping mechanisms every day.

When dealing with depression, I advise using many, if not all, of the coping mechanisms and approaches listed below. It's vital to understand that because sadness typically saps motivation, you probably won't be motivated to accomplish any of them at first. In other words, be aware that feeling unmotivated until you're halfway through is common. Consider the brighter side of things, which is being alive and knowing that you can and will battle this.

1. Intent: Look for tiny ways to help others.

Find personal fulfillment by contributing to a cause greater than yourself. Bear in mind that service need not be extensive to be valued. Think about it: Success, like happiness, cannot be sought for; it must happen naturally. As the unanticipated result of one's personal commitment to a goal bigger than them.

2. Your objectives: Choose realistic objectives that make you feel successful.

When discussing objectives, the majority of people feel bad because their goals are illogical or unattainable. A goal is feasible if:

a. Something that is under your control and independent of others

b. Controllable (i.e., not overwhelming)

c. Suitable for you (not for someone else)

d. Quantifiable (i.e., you know whether or not it is done or getting done)

Instead of adopting a critical, "this is why I'm bad," or gloomy attitude when something goes wrong with your objective, ask yourself, "What can I learn from this?" Be cautious when evaluating your progress in comparison to others. We frequently contrast our greatest flaw with another person's greatest strength. It's unjust (and usually not accurate anyhow).

3. Pleasant Activities: Plan enjoyable activities or events.

Do not wait till you are "in the mood." For instance, permit yourself to take a daily 30-minute "holiday" or plan a good hobby. Just bear in mind that you should approach these things with the proper mindset. Practice gratitude as well, by pausing to reflect on what went right rather than just what went wrong today. Think about keeping a notebook of thankfulness. Recognize that acknowledging your blessings does not require you to ignore your challenges.

4. Engagement: Focus on the here and now.

Sometimes, this method is referred to as mindfulness. Try your hardest during activities not to be self-critical of yourself. Although you might not be able to stop the self-criticism, you can recognize it and gently refocus on the here and now. According to research, those who value or are confident in themselves more also have higher levels of self-compassion.

5. Workout and eat healthily.

Your mood can be significantly improved by engaging in moderate exercise five times each week for 30 minutes each session. When exercising at a moderate intensity, it becomes challenging to sing from the diaphragm. Pay attention to how the foods and beverages you are consuming affect your mood. You don't have to follow fad diets, but anyone who regularly binges on carbohydrates, junk food, and energy drinks can experience depression. Keep in mind the benefits of moderation.

6. Relationships: Pay attention to those who uplift you.

Engage in regular conversation with folks that lift you up instead of people that bring you down). While spending some time by yourself is acceptable, try to strike a balance and avoid isolation if you don't want the sadness to last.

7. Get Enough Sleep: Try to maintain a regular sleeping routine.

Achieve equilibrium by getting the right amount of sleep. A surefire method to fuel depression is to stay up late one night and then sleep in a lot the next day. Don't attempt problem-solving late at night when your brain is just partially awake. You're making progress toward beating depression as you use these coping mechanisms.

Antidepressants

Adult clinical depression is the primary indication for the use of antidepressants. They are also used to treat chronic pain and other mental health issues. Adults with moderate to severe depression are typically treated with antidepressants as a first line of defense. They are frequently prescribed in conjunction with talking therapies like CBT (CBT). An approach to problem-solving is used in CBT, a sort of therapy, to help clients' thoughts, moods, and behaviors. According to a study, due to their limited efficacy, antidepressants are not usually advised for treating mild depression.

However, for moderate depression, doctors will occasionally prescribe antidepressants for a few months to see if your symptoms get any better. The medication will be gradually discontinued if you do not experience any improvements during this period.

Typically, a selective serotonin reuptake inhibitor (SSRI), a form of antidepressant, is first prescribed. After around 4 weeks, if your symptoms have not subsided, an alternate antidepressant may be suggested or your dose may be increased. Your general practitioner can prescribe many antidepressants, but some varieties can only be administered under a mental health professional's supervision. If antidepressants alone are ineffective in treating depression, alternative therapies like CBT may be employed to assist in getting better outcomes. They might also administer greater dosages of the drug. First, a course of psychotherapy (talking therapy) that lasts for at least three months should be made available to children and young people with moderate to severe depression. In some situations, fluoxetine, an SSRI, may be prescribed along with psychotherapy to treat moderate to severe depression in young individuals between the ages of 12 and 18. When patients invent an excuse as to why they are unable to do these tasks, depression is more likely to persist. The key to treating depression, regardless of the medicine you're taking, is to engage in several of these activities every day, even when you don't feel like it. Although developing these healthy coping mechanisms may take some time and effort, if we don't make the effort to be healthy today, subsequent "unwellness" may be thrust upon us.

Anxiety

An anxiety response to cancer is common. A cancer diagnosis, cancer treatment, waiting for test results, going through a cancer screening test, or expecting a cancer recurrence can all cause anxiety. Cancer-related anxiety may worsen pain perception, impair sleep, cause nausea and vomiting, and negatively impact the patient's (and their family's) quality of life. Normal anxiety may require its own therapy if it progresses to extremely high distress, becomes disabling, or involves excessive fear or worry. In that case, anxiety might even be linked to lower rates of cancer survival if left untreated. Cancer patients may notice that their anxiety levels rise or fall at different periods. As cancer progresses or treatment intensity increases, a patient may experience increased anxiety. The degree of anxiety felt by one cancer patient may not be the same as the level felt by another. Learning more about their cancer and the treatment they can anticipate can usually help patients feel less anxious. Feelings of anxiety may become overpowering and interfere with cancer therapy for some patients, especially those who had episodes of severe anxiety prior to their cancer diagnosis. Patients with a history of anxiety disorders or depression, as well as those who are dealing with these diseases at the time of diagnosis, are more likely to experience the intense anxiety associated with cancer therapy. Patients who have a history of significant physical or psychological trauma, are in excruciating pain, are incapacitated, have few friends or family members to care for them, have cancer that is not responding to treatment, or have any of these conditions may also have anxiety. Metastases to the central nervous system and lung tumors might result in physical issues that make people anxious. Many cancer drugs and therapies can make you feel more anxious. Contrary to popular belief, people with advanced cancer frequently experience anxiety owing to fears related to uncontrolled pain, being alone, or being dependent on others, rather than fear of dying. Treatment is an effective way to reduce several of these problems.

An anxiety disorder is a specific kind of mental illness. If you suffer from an anxiety disorder, you could experience fear and dread in response to particular things and circumstances. In addition, anxiety can cause bodily symptoms like perspiration and a racing heart. The presence of some anxiety is common. When you receive a new cancer diagnosis, have to deal with a challenge at work, attend an interview, take an exam, or make a significant choice, you might experience anxiety or nervousness. And even good things can come from anxiety. For instance, anxiety helps us focus our attention and makes us aware of potentially dangerous circumstances, keeping us safe.

However, an anxiety disorder goes beyond the normal trepidation and mild fear you might experience occasionally. There is an anxiety condition when:

• Your ability to perform daily activities is effected by anxiety.

• When anything makes you feel something, you frequently overreact.

• You have no influence over how you react to the current state of medicine.

It can be difficult to get through your daily activities if you have an anxiety disorder. Thankfully, there are a number of efficient treatments available for anxiety disorders.

Who is susceptible to anxiety conditions?

An individual's chance of acquiring anxiety disorders may increase due to a combination of genetic and environmental variables. If you have experienced or have ever experienced:

• Some personality qualities, such as shyness or behavioral inhibition, which cause a person to feel uneasy among strangers and steer clear of uncomfortable circumstances.

• Traumatic or stressful experiences as a young kid or adult.

• Anxiety or other mental health issues run in the family.

• A few health ailments, such as thyroid issues and heart arrhythmias (unusual heart rhythms).

Women are more likely to develop anxiety disorders than their male counterpart. Why that occurs is still being investigated by researchers. It could be a result of a woman's hormones, particularly if they change during the month. Men have higher levels of the hormone testosterone, which may help with anxiety. It's also possible that because women are less inclined to seek help, their anxiety gets worse.

Why do anxiety disorders occur?

Like other types of mental illness, anxiety disorders are debilitating. They are not caused by character defects, personal weaknesses, or issues with upbringing. But the exact cause's source of anxiety problems is unknown. A number of variables are at play:

• Chemical imbalance: Prolonged or severe stress can alter the chemical equilibrium that governs your mood. An anxiety disorder might develop if you are under a lot of stress for an extended length of time.

• Environmental factors: Having a traumatic experience might set off an anxiety condition, especially in people who were already predisposed to it genetically.

• Heredity: There is a hereditary component to anxiety problems. Like eye color, they may be inherited from one or both parents.

Signs of anxiety

Each sort of anxiety disorder has a specific symptom that distinguishes it from the rest. The following are general signs of an anxiety disorder:

Physiological signs

• Cold or perspiring hands.

• Mouth ache.

• Palpitations in the heart.

• Nausea.

• Tingling sensations or numbness in the hands or feet.

• Tense muscles.

• Breathing problems.

Mental health issues:

• Sensing anxiety, terror, and unease.

• Nightmares.

• Past memories or flashbacks of the traumatizing event.

• Constant, intrusive thoughts

Behavioral signs

- The inability to remain quiet and steady.

- Ritualistic actions, such as repeatedly washing your hands.

- Sleep issues.

Anxiety management

Some people may have already gone through periods of severe anxiety due to circumstances unrelated to their cancer. The strain of receiving a cancer diagnosis may cause certain anxiety problems to return or worsen. Extreme fear, difficulty understanding information provided by caregivers, or failure to complete treatment are all possible side effects for patients. A doctor may inquire about the symptoms of a patient in order to prepare treatment for their anxiety.

- Have you had any of the following signs or symptoms while receiving cancer treatment? How many days before the start of the treatment, at night, or at any time, and how long do these symptoms last?

- Do you experience anxiety, jitters, or trembling?

- Have you ever experienced tension, fear, or apprehension?

• Have you ever had to stay away from particular situations or activities out of fear?

• Have you experienced a racing or pounding heart?

• Have you ever felt anxious and had problems breathing?

•Have you ever trembled or perspired unnecessarily?

• Have you ever experienced an upset stomach?

• Have you ever had a lump in the throat?

• Do you frequently pace?

• Do you avoid going to sleep at night for fear of passing away while you sleep?

• Do you stress out weeks in advance over the outcomes of the upcoming diagnostic test?

• Has a sudden fear of losing control or going wild struck you?

• Has a sudden fear of passing away struck you?

• Do you frequently worry about when and how serious your pain will get?

• Are you concerned about getting your upcoming painkiller dose in a timely manner?

• Do you stay in bed longer than you should because you worry the pain might get worse if you get up or move around?

• Have you recently felt bewildered or confused?

Adjustment disorder, panic disorder, phobias, generalized anxiety disorder, and anxiety disorders brought on by other common medical illnesses are examples of anxiety disorders. It could be challenging to distinguish between typical cancer-related anxieties and abnormally intense fears that could be indicative of an anxiety disorder. Treatment is based on how the patient's anxiety affects their day-to-day activities. Treatment of the underlying cause usually relieves anxiety that is brought on by pain, another medical condition, a certain kind of tumor, or a side effect of medicine (such as steroids). It is frequently beneficial to work together with your oncologist and a psychiatrist to detect any anxiety disorders that may be present and to identify any potential interactions between chemotherapy and other medications that may be causing your anxiety symptoms.

Giving the patient the necessary knowledge and support is the first step in treating their anxiety. A patient can reduce anxiety by learning coping mechanisms include viewing their cancer as a problem that has to be solved, learning more about their condition and potential treatments, and utilizing the support systems and resources that are available to them. Patients may gain from additional anxiety treatments, such as psychotherapy,

Group counseling,

Family counseling,

Attending self-help meetings,

Hypnosis, as well as relaxation methods like biofeedback or guided imagery (a type of concentrated concentration on mental images to help with stress management).

The use of medications is optional and can be combined with these methods. In general, patients shouldn't steer clear of anxiety-relieving drugs out of concern for addiction. Their doctors will provide patients just enough medication to get rid of the symptoms, and then they'll start cutting back as the symptoms go away.

How to deal with anxiety disorders effectively

You can take a number of actions to manage the symptoms of an anxiety illness. The following techniques can also help your treatment be more successful:

• Examine stress management: Discover techniques for reducing stress, such as meditation.

• Participate in support groups, which may be found both offline and online. They urge those who suffer from anxiety disorders to talk about their struggles and coping mechanisms.

• Become informed: To feel more in control, educate yourself about the exact sort of anxiety problem you are experiencing. Give your family and friends information about your disease so they can support you.

• Limit or stay away from caffeine: Many individuals with anxiety disorders discover that coffee can exacerbate their symptoms.

• Speak with your healthcare provider; they are a part of your care team. Contact your provider if you think your treatment isn't working or if you have any questions about your medicine. You two can decide how to proceed in the most effective way.

Considerations Following Treatment

A cancer survivor could experience new worries when their cancer treatment is over. Survivors may feel anxious when they return to work and are questioned about their cancer experience or when they run into issues with their insurance. A survivor can be afraid of upcoming follow-up exams and diagnostic testing, or they might be afraid of a cancer recurrence. Survivors may have anxiety as a result of post-traumatic stress, sexual dysfunction, reproductive problems, or changes in their body image. To assist people in readjusting to life after cancer, survivorship programs, support groups, therapy, and other resources are provided.

Delirium

Delirium is a confused state of mind that can happen to cancer patients. The daytime phenomenon could come and go. Delirium is a confused state of mind that can happen to cancer patients, particularly those with advanced cancer. Delirium patients struggle with the following:

• Attention.

• Thinking.

• Awareness.

• Behavior.

• Emotions.

• Judgment.

• Memory.

• Control of muscle.

• Awakening and sleeping.

Delirium comes in three different forms:

• Hypoactive: The patient is inactive and exhibits signs of fatigue, depression, or sleepiness.

• Hyperactive: The patient exhibits agitation or restlessness.

• Mixed: The patient alternates between periods of hypo activity and periods of hyperactivity.

Delirium symptoms typically strike suddenly. They might come and go and frequently happen within a few hours or days. Delirium can be treated and is frequently transient. Delirium, however, may become persistent in the final 24 to 48 hours of life due to issues including organ failure. Most people with advanced cancer experience delirium in the final hours to days before passing away.

Delirium's root causes

• Delirium may be brought on by other medical disorders, cancer, cancer therapy, or both.

• It's critical to understand the causes of delirium.

In cancer patients, there are frequently multiple causes of delirium, particularly when the cancer is advanced and the patient has a number of other medical issues. Delirium can result from the following factors:

• Failure of an organ, such as the liver or kidneys.

• Imbalances in electrolytes: Salt, potassium, calcium, and phosphorus are all essential electrolytes found in blood and other physiological fluids. The heart, kidneys, nerves, and muscles require these electrolytes to function properly.

• Infections.

• Paraneoplastic syndromes: Symptoms that develop when white blood cells or antibodies that fight cancer mistakenly kill healthy nerve cells in the nervous system.

• Drug and treatment side effects: Cancer patients may be prescribed medications that cause delirium and confusion as adverse effects. After the medication is stopped, the side effects typically disappear.

• Withdrawing from drugs that depress the central nervous system (brain and spinal cord).

Danger signs of delirium

Those who have cancer are more prone to experience multiple delirium risk factors. Early detection of risk factors may aid in delirium prevention or shorten the duration of its treatment. The following are risk factors:

• A critical illness.

• Having multiple illnesses.

• Growing old.

• Dementia.

• A low blood protein level called albumin, which is frequently brought on by liver issues.

• Infection.

• High blood levels of nitrogen waste products, which are frequently brought on by kidney issues.

•Using drugs that have mental or behavioral effects.

• Utilizing opioid painkillers in large amounts.

When a patient has multiple risk factors, the risk rises. Hospitalized older cancer patients with advanced disease may have many delirium risk factors.

Delirium's Effects on the Patient, Family, and Healthcare Professionals

• The patient's behavior changes as a result of delirium, upsetting the family and caregivers.

• Communication and physical health may be impacted by delirium.

If delirium impairs the patient's judgment, it could be harmful. Patients with delirium may act in peculiar ways. Even a patient who is quiet or composed can suddenly change their attitude or become upset and require additional attention. Delirium can distress family members and caregivers. Family members frequently assume that an agitated patient is in pain, although this isn't always the case. The family and caregivers may be better able to determine how much pain medication is required if they are aware of the distinctions between the signs of delirium and pain. The family and caregivers can be assisted in learning about these distinctions by health care professionals.

Those that have delirium include:

• More prone to falling.

• Occasionally unable to regulate bowels and/or the bladder.

• More susceptible to dehydration (drink too little water to stay healthy).

Compared to individuals without delirium, they frequently require a lengthier hospital stay. These patients' perplexed mental states could cause them to:

• Being unable to express their wants and feelings to family members and caregivers.

• Incapable of making care-related decisions.

This makes it more challenging for medical professionals to evaluate the patient's symptoms. There may be times when the patient's family must make decisions. Sudden personality changes, difficulty thinking, and unusual worry or depression are also potential delirium warning signs. There are many similarities between the signs of dementia and delirium.

To identify the delirium's underlying causes, doctors utilize physical examinations and other laboratory procedures.

The following symptoms may signal delirium when they appear suddenly:

• Agitation.

• Being uncooperative.

• Variations in personality or conduct.

• Possibilities thinking

• Issues with concentration.

• Unusual depression or anxiousness.

Early signs of delirium resemble those of dementia and depression. When delirium makes a patient sedentary, it can mimic depression. Memory, reasoning, and judgment issues are common in both delirium and dementia. Alzheimer disease is just one of the illnesses that can lead to dementia. The following are some differences between dementia and delirium symptoms:

• Patients with delirium frequently exhibit variations in their level of alertness or awareness. Until their dementia is quite advanced, patients with dementia typically remain conscious and alert.

• Delirium strikes quickly (within hours or days). Dementia develops over months or years and worsens gradually.

Those who have cancer and are older may also have dementia and delirium. The doctor may find it challenging to identify the issue as a result. When delirium is treated yet the symptoms still persist, dementia is more likely to be the cause. Delirium and dementia can be identified by monitoring the patient's condition and symptoms over time.

Doctors will look into delirium's underlying causes through,

• Physical examination and medical history: An examination of the body to check for general health indicators, including looking for disease symptoms like tumors or anything else that seems out of the ordinary. There will also be a history obtained of the patient's health practices, prior diseases, including depression, and treatments. A physical examination can aid in excluding a physical ailment that might be the source of symptoms.

•Laboratory tests are methods used in medicine to examine samples of tissue, blood, urine, or other bodily substances. These tests support disease diagnosis, therapy planning and evaluation, or long-term disease monitoring.

Controlling delirium

Delirium's causes and symptoms can both be managed medically. The following determines how to treat you:

• The patient's residence, such as their home, a medical facility, or a nursing home.

• The stage of the cancer.

• How the patient is being affected by the delirium symptoms.

• The patient's and their family's preferences.

Following are typical treatments for delirium's underlying causes:

• Reducing or stopping the dosage of delirium-inducing medication.

• Fluid administration to treat dehydration

• Pharmacological management of hyperkalemia (too much calcium in the blood).

• Antibiotic in treating infections.

If a patient has delirium and is terminally ill, the doctor might only treat the symptoms. Throughout treatment, the doctor will continue to keep a careful eye on the patient.

Mild delirium symptoms could be helped by managing the patient's environment. The following can be useful:

• Keep the patient's room calm, well-lit, and furnished with familiar items.

• Place a clock or calendar in a visible location for the patient.

• Invite family members to join you.

• As often as you can, stick with the same caregivers.

Physical restrictions may be required for patients who pose a risk of harm to themselves or others.

Medicines may be used in treatment.

Depending on the condition of the patient and the condition of their heart, medication may be used to treat the symptoms of delirium. Because of the dangerous adverse effects of these medications, the patient will be under a doctor's strict observation. The following is a list of these medications:

• Haloperidol.

• Olanzapine.

• Risperidone.

• Lorazepam.

• Midazolam.

Other therapies can be required if the symptoms of delirium are severe, the patient is in pain, or they are having problems breathing. Sometimes, patients will be given medications to sedate (quiet) them. This choice will be jointly made by the family and the medical staff. The following factors may help determine whether to sedate a patient with delirium:

• Before the delirium is deemed resistant (does not respond to treatment), the patient will undergo multiple evaluations by professionals.

Rather than being decided by a single doctor, the choice to sedate the patient is reviewed by a group of medical professionals.

• Before using continuous sedation for brief periods of time, such as overnight, it is taken into consideration

• The medical staff will consult with the family to ensure that they are aware of the team's goals and that they comprehend palliative sedation.

Getting Rid of Delirium

Delirium can be terrifying and lonely, particularly if it is accompanied by troubling ideas, memories, or visions. You might find it beneficial to discuss these with your family, general practitioner, or another healthcare expert. If your problems persist after three months, you should definitely seek medical assistance.

Activities, schedules, and maintaining direction

•Maintain a regular schedule by rising and retiring at the same time every day.

• Always have a calendar or diary on hand to remind you of the day and date. Use these to write down key chores and appointments that you need to remember each day.

• To check the time of day, wear a watch or maintain a clock in the space.

•Make a list of the things you like to do, and pick one from it each day.

• Try solving puzzles, such as crosswords, word searches, and Sudoku's, to keep your mind sharp.

During the day, make an effort to obtain some natural light and fresh air. Sit by a window if you are unable to leave the room.

Make an effort to interact with them in person or over the phone.

Nutritional intake;

Aim for three meals per day.

Decide on meals you enjoy eating.

• Keep up your fluid intake: consistently sip water or other fluids throughout the day (unless advised against this by your doctor).

Hearing and vision

Keep your glasses and hearing aids close at hand so you don't forget to put them on.

Verify whether the batteries in your hearing aids need to be changed.

Sleeping

• Stick to a regular schedule; rise and retire at the same time every day.

•Drink something warm before going to bed, like warm milk or herbal tea.

• Avoid caffeine after 4 o'clock (coffee, tea, etc.).

If you have trouble falling asleep, consider donning an eye mask and some earplugs.

Before going to bed, try some relaxation techniques or listen to music.

Exercise

• Try to exercise every day; if you can't go outside, walk about your house (use a walking aid if needed).

•Think about performing some chair or bed exercises (ask a physiotherapist for advice if needed).

Relaxation

Every day, set aside a designated time for unwinding. Numerous internet resources offer workouts and guided relaxation techniques (see below). Here are a few concepts:

If you have anxiety or have trouble falling asleep, try this exercise:

• Assume a cozy position and check your body temperature.

• Visualize yourself in a tranquil setting, such as a beach, a field covered in wild flowers, or your favorite location.

• Inhale gently via your nose, followed by a calm exhalation. Make effort to breathe in more slowly and deeply. Do this five times.

Another method is progressive muscle relaxation, which involves gradually tensing and relaxing each muscle in your body.

•Sit or lie down in a comfortable posture, and make sure you're warm enough.

• As you inhale, begin by tensing (clenching) the muscles of your toes and feet. As you exhale, completely release them.

When you inhale, contract your leg muscles; as you exhale, completely relax them.

• Tense and relax the muscles in your legs, stomach, arms, hands, shoulders, and face as you work your way up your body.

• Pause for a moment to acknowledge your feelings.

Post-traumatic stress disorder

Anxiety disorders include post-traumatic stress disorder (PTSD). A person may experience PTSD after being exposed to a terrifying or life-threatening circumstance. A horrific event can cause post-traumatic stress disorder (PTSD), a mental health disease that can be brought on by experiencing it or seeing it. Flashbacks, nightmares, excruciating anxiety, and uncontrollable thoughts about the incident are just a few possible symptoms. The majority of people who suffer traumatic circumstances might initially find it hard to adjust and cope, but as time goes on time and by practicing adequate self-care, they typically get better. You may have PTSD if the symptoms worsen, last for weeks, months, or even years, and affect your daily functioning. It can be crucial to seek appropriate treatment after developing PTSD symptoms in order to lessen symptoms and enhance function.

Most frequently, traumatic situations like these are linked to PTSD:

- Contact with combat or violence

- Abuse of children physically

- Sexual assault

- Physical violence

- Receiving a weapon threat

- Natural catastrophe

- A mishap

But it can also happen to cancer patients. For instance, one study found that almost 1 in 4 newly diagnosed breast cancer patients also had PTSD. The following aspects of a cancer event could result in PTSD:

- The findings

- Cancer-related or other bodily discomfort

- Examinations and therapies

- Test outcomes

- Extended hospital stays or procedures

- A recurrence of the cancer or worry of a recurrence

Many patients experience PTSD-like symptoms at first after surviving a horrific cancer incident, such as being unable to stop thinking about what happened. Trauma often causes reactions like fear, anxiety, wrath, depression, and guilt. The majority of trauma survivors do not, however, experience chronic post-traumatic stress disorder. Receiving prompt support and assistance may stop typical stress reactions from becoming worse and turning into PTSD. This can entail reaching out to loved ones and close friends who will soothe you and listen. It can entail contacting a mental health expert for a brief course of therapy. It could be beneficial for some persons to seek aid from their religious group. Support from others may also help you avoid using unhealthy coping mechanisms like abusing alcohol or drugs.

Risk factors

Any age group can suffer from post-traumatic stress disorder. The precise trauma that sets off cancer-related post-traumatic stress disorder isn't usually known to a patient suffering with cancer. It is considerably more difficult to pinpoint the precise source of stress in the cancer experience than it is in other traumas, such natural disasters or rape. The following things, however, could increase your risk of developing PTSD after a traumatic event:

• Suffering from severe or protracted trauma

• Having already gone through trauma, such as losing a loved one to cancer;

• Working in the healthcare industry or having a career that involves the healthcare system increases your chance of being exposed to traumatic occurrences.

• Suffering from other mental health issues, such as depression or anxiety

• Having substance abuse issues, such as problems with excessive drinking or drug usage

• Not having a strong network of family and friends to lean on

• Having biological relatives who experience anxiety or sadness or other mental health issues

Symptoms

Post-traumatic stress disorder symptoms typically occur within the first three months following the incident, although they can also take months or even years to manifest. Therefore, long-term monitoring is necessary for cancer survivors and their families. Some persons who have experienced a traumatic event may exhibit early symptoms but not full-blown PTSD. Patients with these early symptoms frequently go on to develop PTSD, nevertheless. Repeated screenings and close monitoring should be given to these individuals and their family members.

Intrusive memories, avoidance, unfavorable changes in thought and attitude, and changes in bodily and emotional reactions are the four main categories of PTSD symptoms. The severity of symptoms can change over time or from person to person.

Intrusive memories

These are some signs of intrusive memories:

• Constant, frightening flashbacks of the cancer event

• Acting as though the chemotherapy experience just occurred again (flashbacks)

• Recurrent nightmares or disturbing dreams concerning the distressing incident

• Extreme emotional distress or physical repercussions when something brings up the unpleasant experience.

Avoidance

Avoidance symptoms could include:

• Attempting to avoid contemplating or discussing chemotherapy

• Steering clear of situations, people, and places that bring up memories of your cancer or chemo treatment

Negative shifts in attitude and thought

Negative shifts in thought and mood might manifest as the following symptoms:

• Negative perceptions of oneself, others, or the world.

• Lack of optimism for the future

• Memory issues, such as forgetting crucial details about cancer and cancer treatments.

• Trouble keeping tight ties.

• Feeling cut off from friends and family

• A lack of interest in once-enjoyed activities

• Difficulty feeling happy feelings

• Sensing emotional numbness

Alterations in physiological and emotional responses

Arousal symptoms, often known as altered bodily and emotional responses, might include:

• Easily startled or terrified

• Being vigilant at all times when attending a follow-up appointment.

• Self-destructive conduct, such as binge drinking or speeding

• Restless nights

• Difficulty concentrating

• Anger, irritability, or violent behavior

• Extreme humiliation, guilt, or disappointment

Signs and symptoms for kids aged 6 and under may also include:

• Using play to reenact the chemotherapy event or specifics of the cancer occurrence

• Terrifying dreams that may or may not feature chemo event details

The severity of PTSD symptoms might change over time. When you are generally stressed out or come across memories of what you went through, you may have greater PTSD symptoms.

Controlling PTSD

Post-traumatic stress disorder has substantial, long-lasting effects. It might make it difficult for the patient to lead a typical life and might have an impact on their personal connections, education, and employment. The patient may put off receiving medical attention because post-traumatic stress includes avoiding locations and people associated with cancer.

Cancer survivors must be aware of the potential mental anguish associated with having the disease and the importance of receiving prompt post-traumatic stress disorder treatment. There may be more than one type of treatment used. Treatment for post-traumatic stress disorder might assist you in regaining control over your life. Although medicines may also be used, psychotherapy is the main form of treatment. Combining these therapies can help your symptoms go better by:

• Giving you the tools to deal with your symptoms

• Improving your perspective on the world, others, and yourself

• Developing coping mechanisms in case any symptoms recur.

• Addressing other issues that are frequently correlated with cancer experiences, such as alcohol or drug abuse, depression, or anxiety

You don't have to make an effort to manage the effects of PTSD by yourself.

Psychotherapy

Various forms of psychotherapy, commonly known as talk therapy, can be used to treat PTSD in both adults and children. One example of a psychotherapy modality used to treat PTSD is:

Cognitive rehabilitation you can identify the cognitive patterns (ways of thinking) that are holding you stuck with the use of this sort of talk therapy. Patients may benefit from cognitive behavioral treatment (CBT) in the following ways:

• Recognize their symptoms.

• Acquire skills in stress management and coping (such as relaxation training).

• Recognize distress-inducing thought patterns and replace them with more healthy and practical ways of thinking.

• Lessen your sensitivity to distressing triggers.

Cognitive therapy is frequently used with exposure therapy for PTSD.

Exposure treatment

This behavioral therapy supports you in securely confronting memories and events that make you feel uncomfortable so you can develop appropriate coping mechanisms. Flashbacks and nightmares may respond particularly well to exposure therapy. One method involves using virtual reality applications that let you return to the scene of your trauma.

Eye movement desensitization and reprocessing (EMDR).

You can process painful memories and alter how you respond to them with the use of EMDR, which combines exposure therapy and a series of guided eye movements.

Your therapist can assist you in learning stress management techniques so that you can deal with stress in your life more effectively. All of these methods can assist you in taking charge of lingering fear following a traumatic occurrence. Your mental health professional and you can talk about what kind of counseling or treatment options would best suit your requirements.

Try group treatment, individual counseling, or both. A way to interact with people going through comparable circumstances is through group therapy.

Medications

Several different kinds of drugs can aid in reducing PTSD symptoms:

• Antidepressants. These drugs can help with anxiety and depression symptoms. They can also aid in enhancing attention and sleep issues. The Food and Drug Administration (FDA) has granted SSRI approval for the treatment of PTSD for the drugs paroxetine (Paxil) and sertraline (Zoloft).

• Medications that treat anxiety. These medications can treat severe anxiety and its related issues. Since some anti-anxiety drugs have the potential for abuse, they are often only taken temporarily.

• Prazosin. A more recent study found no advantage over a placebo, despite multiple studies suggesting that prazosin (Minipress) may lessen or suppress nightmares in some PTSD sufferers.

If someone is thinking about using prazosin, they should consult a medical professional to see if their specific circumstances would justify trying the medication.

Together, you and your doctor may choose the drug that will treat your symptoms and situation the best and have the fewest adverse effects. Within a few weeks, your mood and other symptoms may start to improve. Inform your doctor of any prescription side effects or issues. Before finding the correct prescription for you, you might need to try more than one, a combination of medications, or your doctor might need to change your dosage or schedule.

Trying to overcome PTSD

A mental health expert or your doctor should be consulted if a chemotherapy event affects your life. As you continue receiving post-traumatic stress disorder treatment, you can additionally do the following things:

• Adhere to your treatment schedule. Even though it could take some time for therapy or medicine to start working, most patients do recover. Keep in mind that it takes time. You can advance if you stick to your treatment plan and keep in regular contact with your mental health expert.

• Get to know PTSD. When you have a better understanding of how you're feeling, you may create coping mechanisms that will enable you to react appropriately.

• Look after yourself. Get enough sleep, maintain a nutritious diet, engage in exercise, and relax. Caffeine and nicotine should be limited or avoided as they might make anxiety worse.

• Avoid self-medication. It may be tempting to use drink or drugs to dull your emotions, but doing so is unhealthy. It may cause additional issues in the future, obstruct curative therapies, and hinder true recovery.

• Stop this cycle. Take a quick stroll or dive into a hobby to help you refocus when you're feeling stressed.

• Maintain contact. Spend time with people who are encouraging and caring, such as family, friends, religious leaders, or others. If you don't want to, you are under no obligation to discuss what took place. Even just spending time with loved ones can be therapeutic and consoling.

• Give support groups some thought. Find a support system by contacting your local social services agency, or a mental health professional. Alternatively, search a directory of local support groups online.

When a loved one suffers from PTSD

The person you love could appear to be a different person than the one you knew before chemotherapy, such as withdrawn and despondent or angry and irritated. The emotional and mental health of friends and family members who have PTSD may be severely strained. It could be tough for you to learn about the trauma that chemotherapy caused and that resulted in your loved one developing PTSD. It might even bring up painful memories for you. If your loved one tries to talk about the trauma, you may find yourself avoiding them or losing faith in their ability to recover. You could feel terrible that you can't help your loved one get better or hasten the healing process at the same time. Keep in mind that nobody can be changed. You can, however.

• Get to know PTSD. This can aid in your understanding of what your loved one is experiencing.

•Realize that withdrawal and avoidance are symptoms of the disease. If your loved one refuses your help, give them some space and let them know you're there for them when they're ready to receive it.

• Offer to go to doctor's visits. Attending appointments, if your loved one is willing, can aid in understanding and supporting therapy.

• Be ready to pay attention. Let your loved one know that you are available to listen but that you respect his or her decision not to speak. Avoid pressuring your loved one to discuss the experience before they are prepared.

Encourage involvement and plan out times to spend with friends and family. Make your personal health a priority. By eating well, exercising regularly, and getting enough sleep, you can take good care of yourself. Spend time alone or with companions engaging in rejuvenating activities.

If you need assistance, get it. Consult your doctor if you're having trouble handling things. He or she might suggest a therapist who can assist you in managing your stress.

Stay secure. If your loved one starts to act violently or abusively, prepare a secure spot for you and your kids to go.

Getting ready for the appointment

Make an appointment with your doctor or a mental health expert if you believe you may have post-traumatic stress disorder. You can use the following details to help you get ready for your appointment and know what to expect. If you can, bring a dependable family member or friend. It might occasionally be challenging to recall all the information that has been given to you.

How you can help

Make the following list before your appointment:

• Any symptoms you've had and how long you've had them.

• Important details about you, particularly incidents or encounters from your recent past that left you feeling terribly scared, helpless, or horrified. If there are memories you can't immediately access without having a strong need to put them out of your mind, your doctor will benefit from knowing this.

• Activities you've quit doing or are staying away from due to stress.

• Details about your health, such as any additional physical or mental illnesses you may have been prescribed. Include the names and amounts of any vitamins or drugs you are taking.

Questions to ask in order to maximize your appointment.

Asking your doctor or a mental health expert the following fundamental questions could be helpful:

What, in your opinion, is the root of my symptoms?

Are there any further potential causes?

•How will you make a diagnosis for me?

Is my condition likely to be short-term or chronic?

What therapies would you suggest for this disorder?

I have additional health issues. How can I handle them and my PTSD the best?

• When do you anticipate that my symptoms will go better?

Does having PTSD make me more likely to develop other mental health issues?

•Do you suggest making any adjustments at work, home, or school to promote recovery?

• Would telling my coworkers or professors about my diagnosis aid in my recovery?

Do you have any printed resources on PTSD that I might borrow? What websites would you suggest?

During your appointment, do not be afraid to inquire about anything else.

What to anticipate from your physician

You might anticipate a number of inquiries from your doctor. Be prepared to respond so that you can set aside time to discuss any points you want to emphasize. Your doctor might query:

• Which signs worry you or your family members?

When did you or your loved ones notice your symptoms for the first time?

Have you ever been involved in or seen a distressing event?

Are you still having unsettling dreams, recollections, or thoughts related to the trauma you underwent?

•Do you avoid particular individuals, locations, or circumstances that make you think back on the traumatic event?

Do you currently have challenges at work, school, or in your personal relationships?

• Have you ever considered harming yourself or someone else?

Do you consume alcohol or use drugs for fun? How often?

•Have you ever undergone treatment for mental illness or other psychiatric symptoms? If so, which therapy was the most beneficial?

Multiple pain syndromes.

The impact of a physiological chain of electrical and chemical events taking place in the body is what is referred to as "pain."

Pain is an unpleasant sensory and emotional experience connected with existing or potential tissue damage or explained in terms of such damage, claims the International Association for the Study of Pain. Cancer patients endure pain at many locations throughout their bodies, which can have a variety of causes and symptoms. Cancer pain can be minor or severe, short-lived or long-lasting. One or more organ systems, bones, or organ systems may be impacted.

According to research, between 30 and 50 percent of cancer patients will endure pain during their treatments. On the other hand, a staggering 70 to 90% of individuals with advanced cancer endure episodes of agony. Patients with cancer have certain common pain pathways. These include tissue degeneration, infection-related inflammation, and obstruction of hollow organs, tissue degradation, and tumor formation in constrained areas with an abundance of pain receptors.

Most cancer pain syndrome patients experience increased pain as a result of their lack of awareness and control over their condition. It's crucial for individuals with cancer pain syndromes to understand that they have a completely legal right to effective pain management. They must understand the following:

Most discomfort is manageable.

Communication is crucial.

•Pain can be quantified.

Patients and healthcare professionals can collaborate to effectively manage pain.

Cancer types and pain

Nociceptive pain and neuropathic pain are the two main types of pain that a person with cancer pain syndromes typically feels

Nociceptive Pain

This kind of pain is brought on by tissue injury and is frequently described as being acute, agonizing, or throbbing. The bodily parts close to the cancer site get crowded with tumors or cancer cells, which causes nociceptive pain. This discomfort may also be brought on by cancer that has spread to the bones, muscles, or joints.

Neuropathic Pain

Actual nerve injury results in this kind of pain. A tumor pressing against a nerve or a group of nerves may cause it. People who are feeling this kind of cancer pain frequently describe it as a scorching, heavy, or even numbing sensation.

Pain's Origins

There are numerous potential sources of discomfort for a patient with cancer pain syndrome. The most crucial of these is:

• Suffering from tumor pain

Most often, cancer pain results from a tumor pressing against a bone, a nerve, or an organ. The location may also influence the pain. For instance, a small tumor next to a nerve or the spinal cord may cause excruciating agony. On the other hand, a larger tumor somewhere else might not be as painful.

Pain from cancer treatment

Another source of discomfort is medical procedures, including surgery, radiation, and chemotherapy. Pain is another side effect that many patients experience as a result of their medicines' suppressed immune systems.

• Others

It's possible that other factors have nothing to do with your particular disease. Examples of these include migraines, strained muscles, arthritis, kidney stones, a herniated disk in the back, and other conditions.

Treatment of the multiple pain syndrome

Effective management of the cancer pain syndrome can be achieved by carefully balancing pharmacological and non-pharmacological therapies.

Pharmaceutical therapy

The most common drugs used to manage pain are listed here along with some examples.

Acetaminophen, aspirin, and ibuprofen are non-opioids.

• Opioids: Fentanyl, Hydromorphone, Hydrocodone, Hydromorphone, and Morphine

• Amitriptyline, imipramine, doxepin, and trozoldone are antidepressants.

• Gabapentin, an antiepileptic drug

• Dexamethasone and Prednisone are steroids.

Other treatments comprise:

• Radiation treatment

• Nerve blocks/pump implants

• Neurosurgery

• Surgery

Non pharmacological therapy

The primary natural remedies are as follows:

- Biofeedback

- Relaxation and breathing exercises

- Distraction

- Hot and cold packs and heating pads

- Hypnosis

- Imagery

- Pressure, vibration, and massage

- Transcutaneous Electrical nerve stimulation (TENS)

- Rest

Medication use

The majority of medications used for this purpose are taken orally in the form of liquid or tablets. Patients who are unable to take the drug in this way occasionally have other options as well, such as:

- Rectal suction devices

- Topical patches

Injections (Subcutaneous, Intravenous, Epidural, Sub dermal and Intramuscular)

Overcoming multiple pain syndrome

You could feel irate, depressed, despondent, or despair when you're in pain. Your personality may change, your sleep may be disturbed, and your work and relationships may be affected by pain. In turn, stress, sleep deprivation, depression, and anxiety can all exacerbate pain. By lowering the high levels of physiological stress that frequently exacerbate pain; psychological treatment offers secure, drug-free techniques that can relieve your pain directly. By teaching you how to deal with the numerous issues linked to pain, psychological counseling also helps to lessen the indirect effects of pain.

Education plays a significant role in psychological pain treatment; it provides patients with the tools they need to deal with a highly challenging issue.

In the past ten years, acupuncture, mind-body therapies, and various dietary supplements have helped a lot of patients find pain relief. Others utilize therapeutic touch, massage, chiropractic, and osteopathic (bone) manipulation therapies, as well as some herbal treatments and dietary regimens, to reduce pain. However, there is little to no scientific proof to back up these pain relieving techniques.

Treatments known as mind-body therapies are designed to support the body's capacity to influence how the mind feels and behaves. Diverse techniques are employed in mind-body therapy, including hypnosis, guided imagery, meditation, relaxation techniques, and biofeedback. Relaxation methods can ease discomfort brought on by chronic pain. The use of visualization might be a useful additional pain-relieving strategy. Try the following exercise: Try to visualize the pain by closing your eyes and giving it a shape, color, size, and motion. Try gradually changing this image to one that is more aesthetically pleasant, harmonic, and smaller. Another strategy is to keep a journal of your pain experiences as well as the contributing and mitigating circumstances. Examine your journal frequently to look for potential areas for change. Try to see suffering as a necessary but limited aspect of existence.

By letting you know how your muscle tension affects your pain, electromyography (EMG) biofeedback can teach you how to manage it. Through refocusing techniques, hypnotherapy, and self-hypnosis, may assist you in blocking or transforming pain. Glove anesthesia is a self-hypnosis technique that involves entering a trance, laying a hand over the painful location, visualizing the hand as relaxed, heavy, and numb, and visualizing these sensations as taking the place of other, unpleasant feelings in the affected area.

Meditation

When used frequently, relaxation methods like yoga and meditation have been demonstrated to lessen discomfort brought on by stress. Yoga's mild stretches are especially effective at building muscles without adding to overall physical stress.

Acupuncture

By stimulating the release of endorphins, which are molecules that inhibit pain, acupuncture is supposed to lessen discomfort. Numerous acupoints are close to nerves. These nerves generate a dull discomfort or a sensation of being overly full in the muscle when activated. Endorphins are released when the central nervous system (the brain and spinal cord) receives a signal from the activated muscle, preventing the brain from receiving a pain signal.

Numerous pain-related illnesses, such as headaches, low back pain, menstrual cramps, carpal tunnel syndrome, tennis elbow, fibromyalgia, osteoarthritis (particularly of the knee), and myofascial pain, may benefit from acupuncture as a complementary therapy. A comprehensive pain treatment program could also incorporate acupuncture as an option or as a component of it.

Massage and Chiropractic Treatment

The most popular non-surgical back pain treatment is chiropractic care. In several trials, those who received chiropractic adjustments showed improvements. However, the majority of scientific trials have failed to provide strong evidence for the treatment's ability to effectively cure chronic back and neck pain. The effectiveness of chiropractic treatment for the management of cancer pain is now being evaluated by more studies.

Fighting cancer

Researchers are currently working on ways to actively involve the mind in the body's fight against cancer by employing practices like visualization, biofeedback, and meditation (creating in the mind positive images of what is occurring in the body). Some medical professionals and psychologists now think that having the right mindset might even directly affect cell activity, which can therefore be used to stop, if not completely cure, cancer. The focus of this emerging scientific discipline, known as psychoneuroimmunology, is on how mental and emotional activity affects physical health, suggesting that patients can have a much more significant impact on their recovery.

We won't know whether the immunological defense system can be controlled by the mind for many years. Biofeedback and visualization experiments are beneficial because they promote optimistic thinking and relaxation, which boosts one's will to live. However, if a patient places all of his or her trust in them and disregards traditional therapy, they may also be harmful.

The Mind's Ability

There has been much discussion about the role of the mind in both producing and treating sickness. There is a lot of speculation, especially when it comes to cancer. However, unlike what many patients believe, no research has demonstrated in a way that is scientifically valid that a person can control the course of their cancer with their thoughts. The effectiveness of optimistic attitudes and emotions has been demonstrated in numerous particular instances. At the age of 25, a high-risk cancer patient underwent a hysterectomy. At age 31, she was diagnosed with aggressive Stage IV cancer that had spread throughout her liver and bones and had metastasized extensively to her lungs. She also has a remarkable will to live. She once remarked, "I would get out of bed every morning as if nothing were amiss. Although I may have known I would eventually have to confront my problems and that I could feel ill during the day, I never got out of bed that way. I was fighting for many things. I had a lovely life; a three-year-old child, and a mystical relationship with my spouse. She is still alive, receiving chemotherapy, and leading a full life thirty years later.

We frequently ask our patients to describe their ability to overcome their issues. We have discovered that regardless of their differences in age, education level, ethnic or cultural background, or type of disease, they have all undergone a similar process of psychological rehabilitation. All of them consciously choose "to live." After experiencing initial devastation, they simply chose to evaluate their new situation and make the most of each day.

Their "will to live" refers to their strong desire to survive, regardless of their level of fear of passing away. They want to enjoy life; they want to wring more value out of it; they think their life is not done, and they are prepared to do whatever it takes to do that. Our understanding of the value of life, love, friendship, and all that is enjoyable is frequently renewed when death is a possibility. We become more receptive to new opportunities and start taking chances we previously lacked the courage to do. According to a lot of patients, embracing the uncertainties that come with having a disease gives life more purpose. The simplest joys are enhanced, and much of life's hypocrisy is removed. There is still room for joy when resentment and fury start to fade.

"I adore life, and I love nature." Being outside, sensing the sun on my skin or the breeze against my body, listening to birds sing, and inhaling ocean spray I never give up hope that I will come across or be blessed with a victory over this illness.

Building Up Your Will to Live

Unfortunately, and rather unfortunately, a lot of patients view a cancer diagnosis as a death sentence in the same way that individuals in prehistoric cultures saw the imposition of a curse or spell. The "bone pointing" phenomenon generates a paralyzing terror that makes the person just withdraw from society and wait for death to come. Similar phenomena can happen in modern medicine when a patient, out of ignorance or superstition, thinks that being told they have cancer means they will die. The phenomenon of self-willed death, however, only works if the victim has faith in the curse's ability to work its magic. Patients who failed their initial round of chemotherapy treatment for cancer, failed again after their second and third treatments, and then—with more advanced disease—a fourth treatment was quite effective. In order to succeed, obtain remission, or recover with the best quality of life, you must take a risk in everything. Just being willing to take a chance tends to inspire optimism and a favorable environment, which strengthens the elements of the desire to live. There are numerous additional methods for boosting one's will to life. Participating in The finest thing a patient can do to improve their will to live is to actively participate in their own treatment. Patients who approach their illness in a combative manner are no longer seen as helpless victims. Instead, they take an active role alongside their medical support team in the quest for a cure, remission, or improvement. Honesty, open communication, shared responsibility, and education regarding the nature of the disease, treatment options, and rehabilitation must be the cornerstones of this partnership. This partnership leads to an improvement in coping skills, which in turn strengthens the will to live.

Giving and Receiving from Others - Extending the partnership to others is one way to make it stronger. Your love of life and determination to survive are supported by the emotional experience of sharing and enjoying your family and relationships. One of the most crucial insights you come to as you transform from a helpless victim to an activist is that how other people see and treat you has everything to do with you. Others won't feel sorry for you if you can accept your condition and resist feeling sorry for yourself. They'll react in kind without hesitation or awkwardness if you can talk about your illness and medical treatment in an honest manner. You have the power. By being open and honest about what you want to talk about or not talk about as well as being clear about whether and when you need their assistance, you can quietly and softly put your family, friends, and coworkers at rest. Your capacity to cope will improve and you'll be better able to fight for your life if you share your life with others and get help or support from friends and family. A lonely or lonely person frequently feels like a helpless victim. There is a need to talk about your own issues, but assisting others in solving their issues or managing their everyday struggles offers both the giver and the recipient strength. Helping someone in need is one of life's more fulfilling experiences.

Additionally, patients can participate in group therapy or private counseling as part of psychological support programs. The sensation of loneliness, anxiety, and despair that cancer patients frequently experience can often be alleviated by venting complaints to others in comparable situations.

Those who must endure cancer can live as fully as possible by

• focusing on the now rather than the past,

• being open to compromise and establishing reasonable aims;

• reclaiming control over their lives and continuing to feel independent and confident in themselves;

• attempting to overcome depressive thoughts and feelings by actively helping others and oneself; and

• improving one's nutrition and engaging in frequent exercise.

Nurturing Hope

Hope is the most essential component of the will to live. The mental and emotional state of hope is what drives you to continue living, make progress, and be successful. Lack of hope can cause a person to lose the desire to live and give up on life. There is not much to live for without hope. But with hope, it is possible to keep a positive outlook, to be more determined, to have better coping mechanisms, and to be more open to giving and receiving love and support.

Even if a diagnosis makes the future appear bleak, hope must be kept alive. People must rely on hope to survive. Depression arises when you take away hope since you no longer have a chance for the future. People's bodies just shut down when they reach that low emotional state.

As long as there is even a slim prospect of survival, hope can be maintained. It can be sparked by slight improvements or a remission, fostered, and kept alive when crises or reversals happen. There may be moments when you feel worn out and depleted by seemingly endless issues and are prepared to give up the fight for survival. Too sometimes, it appears easier to give up than to continue battling. Sometimes, frustrations and hopelessness can seem insurmountable. Fighting for your health is a demanding endeavor that requires tenacity or unwavering persistence.

Cancer is not only physically harmful, but it can also have a significant negative impact on your battling spirit and will to live. However, even in the most trying circumstances, there are frequently untapped sources of physical and emotional strength that can be called upon to help you get through another day. These reserves can give your life more purpose and act as a lighthouse to guide you through a storm to safety. For every individual, hope means something different. It is a part of having a good attitude and accepting our lot in life. We succeed by utilizing our strengths so that we can fully experience life. Our hopes for happiness, a cure, remission, or a longer lifespan are frequently limited by external factors. We also worry about being poor, hurt, dying horribly, or going through other unpleasant things.

You can worry so much that you lose hope and lose sight of the prospect of a recovery. On the other hand, you risk losing sight of reality if you become overly optimistic and self-assured. Balancing your worries and hope is your biggest difficulty. The way we spend our lives feeds our hope. The highest quality of life demands resolving previous issues, disputes, and family turmoil in addition to performing present obligations. There must be closure on issues that have not been settled. There should be new projects started. If the future appears bleak, you can find comfort in knowing that you have taken care of your business and have not burdened your loved ones or others. You can obtain mental tranquility in this way, which will also serve to make you more determined to live. Try to finish what you can every day so that you can feel satisfy that you gave it your best effort.

To increase your happiness in life, be brave, take risks, and be willing to live each day to the fullest. Life can be lived fully till the last breath as long as fear, misery, and pain are under control. Each of us has the ability to live each day a little bit better, but in order to do so; we must concentrate on our purpose and our goals and implement a reasonable daily plan—often amended several times—to help us get there. The will to live is built on these resources. We can only experience the magnificent sentiments of knowing and experiencing the glories of life and appreciate its meanings through active living by using the force of the will to live—nourished by hope.

Daily affirmations and meditation guide.

Dealing with cancer is quite frightening. It introduces a lot of uncertainty into our lives in one way. On the other hand, we also worry that our life might be about to end. The difficulties you encounter are great regardless of whether you are currently battling cancer, a cancer survivor, or a caregiver.

Get this straight away: You don't have to be upbeat all the time. That is totally unrealistic in my opinion. You are free to spend some time feeling sad, angry, or any other strong emotion. Most importantly, you must be able to find a way to express all of your feelings. When things calm down, you may concentrate on your medical care and rehabilitation. During this period, it is preferable to have a good outlook rather than be depressed. I mean, having an optimistic outlook on life makes sense, right?

How to approach cancer with a positive outlook

You should be aware that cancer is a highly serious illness and should not be treated lightly before continuing. You must get the appropriate treatment as soon as possible and seek competent medical advice. Positive thinking and affirmations are only tools to get you through the process; they are not a means of getting over it.

Now, how can you stay sane and positive at the same time? Because our thoughts are so strong, we need to use our subconscious to alter the way we think about things. Many people, whether from our families, our friends, or our coworkers, have self-limiting views that were probably forced onto us when we were young or inadvertently by those same people. When that occurs, we start to limit ourselves and become mired in negative ideas. With the help of affirmations, we can gradually improve by changing the way our minds function.

Here are some strategies to help you maintain your optimism in these trying times.

1. Mix with folks who share your outlook on life.

Although we are aware of peer pressure, we frequently succumb to it. When was the last time you followed a friend's advice and made a poor choice? Yes, I believe that most people have at least one tale to share. We need supportive people in our lives to provide us the much-needed encouragement as we battle cancer. These are the individuals who can provide the cheer you long for and contribute to improving your days. You can face and manage your worries easier when you have a group of loving and encouraging family and friends at your side. They will be there to offer you a shoulder to cry on and to listen to you. Along with being around positive people, other healthy activities include reading insplrational literature and listening to uplifting music. I urge you to look into coloring books. You may find it silly, but I can guarantee you that as you go through them, they will make you very happy and laugh a lot.

2. Get rid of unhealthy relationships.

I got it. You occasionally have relationships like that that you just can't seem to let go of or maybe even don't want to end. But the reality is that toxic individuals prevent you from growing personally, and if you have cancer, you definitely do not want them near you to make your situation much worse. When possible, stay away from these situations, or you can ask one of your supportive groups to serve as a barrier for you. They need to be able to reject it on your behalf and protect you from such unfavorable treatment.

3. Acquiring a slogan and a fresh outlook

Recall how we discussed reprogramming your subconscious earlier? Instead of attempting to alter the circumstances or events that are happening to you, you may modify the way you think by reframing your perspective. The truth is that there are a lot of factors outside of our control that nevertheless have an impact on us, largely because we give them permission to. If we cannot undo what has already occurred, we must learn to deal with and accept it. Refocusing your thoughts can help you get through challenging circumstances. You could now need to take a medicine cocktail daily, for instance. You may change your perspective and say, "Hey, these bright tablets are going to enhance my immune system and make me stronger soon," as opposed to whining about it. If you let yourself get lost in it, this can be a really satisfying aspect of stress management for you. You can create your own mantra or say cancer affirmations at the same time. It helps if you try to picture the result you want and use these affirmations as a roadmap.

This Is a List of the Top Cancer Affirmations That Will Motivate You

I am aware of how difficult your trip is, but never let that discourage you. If we have faith, any of us can do great things. Daily positive affirmations are an excellent technique to focus if you're feeling lost and need something to do it. They function to swap out any negative thoughts for positive ones in your subconscious mind.

To further assist you, you might also wish to purchase your own affirmations worksheet. Don't think twice and start straight now!

• I am gradually beginning to think more kindly.

• Cancer is not the entirety of your life; it is merely one chapter.

• Today is going to be a great day.

• My life is just getting started.

• Cancer is a disease, but my profound source of comfort is unbounded.

•It will all pass.

•I evaluate my success based on my own standards.

•I'm not going to quit.

•Everything in my body is holy, and I'll cherish it now and every day.

• My body has the ability of healing itself.

• I'll be able to picture myself cancer-free.

• I gently distance myself from individuals who have wronged me in the past and forgive them.

• I'm cherished.

• I am lovely and deserving of anything absolutely lovely.

• I have a right to triumph over breast cancer.

• I only draw prosperous, fun, and advantageous conditions.

•I have courage in my heart and mental clarity as I wake up today.

• Every door I open brings advantages and opportunities.

• I'll protect myself from naysayers by being selective about who I discuss my cancer journey with.

- The therapies I use support my body's ability to heal.

- I receive all of my material and spiritual substance from God.

- Today, I make the decision to exude love, joy, and thankfulness.

- I may encounter cancer, but it will not define me; it will merely be a chapter in my life.

- Miracles occur frequently, and cancer is not exempt from its enchantment, so I go with miracles.

- My cells are all content and healing.

- I trust in miracles.

- I'm becoming the possessor of a cancer-beating mindset.

- I'm a person who is strong and competent.

- I encircle myself with light and love.

- Cancer can be classified, staged, and treated; but, my humanity is bound to the enduring mystery that defies classification, boundaries, and mortality.

- I'll live each day to the fullest.

- As the cancer fades and throws itself into oblivion, I pull energy from the universe by using my consciousness.

- I relish living.

- Everyone in my immediate vicinity is peaceful.

- I'm taken care of.

- I'll be able to handle everything life throws at me once I've defeated breast cancer.

- My body is my temple; the divine resides there.

- The battle may have been started by cancer, but I will win.

- I always work to keep my mind clear of unfavorable ideas.

- I have a strong will.

- My attention is on carrying out my purpose for being on this planet. Everything else is all for show.

- I have the freedom to be open and honest about whom I am.

- I am looked up to by those fighting breast cancers as a source of motivation.

- I'm grateful for my friends, family, and tribe. I'm appreciative that this village is behind me.

- I have no trouble thinking positively.

- Everyone has cancer cells; my body is not an exception; it is retraining itself to recognize and get rid of them.

- I heal quickly.

- I'm incredibly proud to call you a friend.

- I only interact with positive individuals.

- I cherish you.

- I am not defined by my illness.

- I respect my need for rest and renewal.

- I have faith that I will be directed to the physicians and therapies that will help me regain my health.

- I am the most skilled healer.

- Life is peaceful, loving, and pleasurable in the globe.

- My heart also grins when I smile.

- I can battle cancer by utilizing the power of visualizing.

• It's okay to feel frightened. I'm about to do something very, incredibly daring, which is why I'm frightened.

•Every morning when I get up, I pray for you.

• Everything that has occurred, is occurring, and will occur in tranquility for me.

• I am discovering that cancer is losing power every day, and I am no longer afraid to live.

• I will only be among those who have faith in my ability to overcome cancer.

•My dreams are not controlled by cancer.

• My health improves every single day.

• Regardless of the symptoms I experience, my health is improving.

•I have courage.

•People consider me to be a fighter.

•I'm becoming a fighter.

•I'm beating this disease.

•It comes naturally to me to maintain my composure under pressure.

•Nothing can take my delight away.

•My body's cells will teach malignant cells how to go back to their original location when they divide.

•I don't have breast cancer.

•My energy levels are over the roof and my excitement is pouring today.

•Both my scars and I will recover.

• I can quickly destroy papers that are piled up and may include the phrase "cancer" both inside of me and around me.

•I'm going to meet the right person for me sooner than I thought.

• Cancer is a small fraction of a great eternity of wellness, and nothing is going to affect my universe.

•I'll always have a good time and get along with the medical staff.

•Thinking positively is all I know.

• I am making daily progress in beating my sickness.

• I let go of the desire to judge myself against others.

• I benefit myself and others by applying all of my experiences and knowledge.

• All of life's advantages are made available to me.

• Cancer simply isn't big enough to control my great life, so I won't let it define me.

• I'm receiving treatment on all fronts, and I'm already seeing results in the future.

• I'm in good health and am living a long life.

• My courage outweighs my fear.

• Good things are coming my way.

• I am grateful for my head, hair, toes, feet, ankles, legs, and knees.

• Love and companionship are all around me.

• I consume wholesome, easily digested food every day.

• I shall be cancer-free of breast.

• It's not necessary for life to be ideal to be wonderful.

• I am grateful for this lovely day and all the possibilities it offers. I'm confident that something positive will occur.

• My pain or discomfort is momentary. Daily, I feel better.

• Genes can be turned on and off, and with my consent, cancer is turned off.

• I let up of my need to win people over.

• I cherish the little things and find comfort in them.

•I am healed, and healing is a state of the heart and mind.

• I'll hone my mental skills.

• I am gorgeous.

• My health is assured, and I can picture a future where cancer will only be a faint shadow of past reflections.

• My unfulfilled dreams will still come true.

• Every day, I rearrange cells and send errant cells into the light.

• Since I am a warrior, I will not give up.

• Being resilient in the face of potentially fatal circumstances comes naturally to me.

• My ability to think positively is developing.

• My loved ones and friends support me.

• While some people may view cancer as a death sentence, I view it as giving my life a colorful narrative with a beautiful resolution.

• I have an amazing family and wonderful friends, which is a blessing.

• My health and vitality are radiant.

• Nothing is insurmountable.

•Every day, my body gets stronger.

• As I am, I am ENOUGH.

• I am appreciative of my physicians and nurses.

• I look after myself well.

• I will use my dreams and my imagination to create a future in which every day will be a triumph over cancer.

• A cancer diagnosis may initially appear to be a significant barrier to happiness, yet every day I continue to experience it.

• God only sends me favorable circumstances.

• I am more loved than I could ever imagine, braver than I believe, and stronger than I realize.

• I have more friends than I could ever dream, which is a blessing.

• I glow brilliantly with excitement.

• I'm kind to both my body and mind.

• I'm getting stronger every day.

• Though my body may have some cancer, my mind does not; delight is an antidote to unhealthy thoughts.

• My diagnosis does not define my femininity. I am a warrior.

• I'm imagining myself on top of a mountain, radiant and unaffected by cancer.

• I am in excellent health and grateful to be alive.

• I can get assistance when I need it.

• I am a warrior.

• I'm considerably stronger now that I've overcome breast cancer.

• I shall overcome this.

• My own personal hero.

• Although some days are harder than others, difficult is not insurmountable.

• Knowing that I have cancer does not affect who I am; I will continue to live with the same zest and enthusiasm that I did the day before.

• The medication I take is fully aware of what my body needs to do to heal itself.

•I'm not only a conqueror.

• I can do no wrong.

• I will continue to advance each day with confidence in spite of the obstacles I encounter.

•God won't ever abandon me.

• I make the decision to accept myself just as I am.

• I've overcome a lot of challenges. I will also survive this.

• The future is not predetermined; with every new idea, I generate my wellness from cancer.

•I beckon tranquility into my heart.

• I'm here for a purpose. Nothing in my life has happened by accident. I am exactly how God created me to be.

• I'm not going to allow anything or anyone stop me.

• I'm getting more certain that I can get through this.

•I'm doing fine.

• I'll continue to live.

• I am positive that I will survive this ordeal.

• I'm not by myself.

• Love is all around me, inside of me, above me, and below me.

• The joy that is about to come is greater than the sorrow I'm currently experiencing.

• I release cancer out with every exhalation, and I heal with every inhalation.

• As I recover and mend, I spend time getting to know my cancer so that, in the future, we won't be rivals but rather admired teammates.

• My internal environment, including my cancer, is not bad. Misguided cells won't scare me; they can be retrained.

• I am not defined by cancer.

•God will act correctly for me because He loves me.

• Positive ideas flood my mind.

• I have emotional self-control.

• I am attractive and feminine.

• While I sleep, my body heals.

• I am powerful. I am a warrior.

• The strongest people are not those who demonstrate strength in front of us but those who win conflicts we know nothing about.

• Although difficult, the effort will be worthwhile.

• Only a small portion of the billions of cells that make up my physical body are affected by cancer, so I'll concentrate on what's best for me.

• I decide to think only good ideas.

• I'll keep trying.

• I never forget to picture myself overcoming breast cancer.

• Wherever I am planted, I flourish. I've never had deeper roots.

• I always have more money than I need to cover my expenses.

• I have the capacity to fully recover.

•I'll defeat cancer.

• I'm committed to overcoming breast cancer.

• I'm not sure how these upcoming few months will go for me, but I'll always stand up for myself.

• The advantageous position is always mine.

• I surround myself with only positive people in my social circle, which will aid in my battle against breast cancer.

• My medical procedures will be successful, and my body will heal completely.

• I am grateful for my complete healing and excellent health.

• I let go of the past and live a tranquil life.

• It's simple for me to picture myself being cancer-free.

Note: Personalize it by calling your name and mentioning the sort of cancer you have.

How do you address a letter of affirmation to yourself?

Examples and suggestions to help you

We are constantly exposed to external voices. We hear people's complaints, messages, and experiences from friends, family, coworkers, and the news, but we hardly ever take the time to listen to ourselves. You can develop a stronger relationship with your inner ideas and dreams as well as understand the effectiveness of affirmations by creating an affirmation letter to yourself.

A letter of affirmation can help you go beyond your daily affirmations by motivating you to be more focused and succinct about what you actually want to accomplish. An excellent way to organize your ideas and boost your confidence is by writing an affirmation letter. Making advantage of writing therapy to express your feelings is a crucial step in self-care. Writing helps you develop and boost your happiness in a similar way as journaling. Consider it a letter of love to yourself.

What is an affirmation letter?

So what is an affirmation letter precisely, and how do you write one? That's what I'll be talking about here, but first, you should be aware that an affirmation letter uses positive phrases to boost your confidence and self-esteem. Even if you don't currently have a specific goal in mind, you can still write one to highlight your individuality and special qualities or to show appreciation for the positive aspects of your life. The basic fact is that an affirmation letter is a positive message that you write to yourself, regardless of how lengthy or short it is or the language you choose. It should be very private and likely not something you share with others.

What kind of affirmation would this be?

A letter that you write and address to yourself is what an affirmation letter is, in its most basic form (although you can do that for others too). You are supposed to write down your thoughts in an affirmation letter. They might be your feelings, your goals, or something you'd like to manifest. Essentially a positive remark, an affirmation can be used to dispel self-sabotaging, restricting beliefs that are getting in the way of your personal growth. It's crucial to be direct, clear, and to the point while writing an affirmation. Here is an illustration I used to help me in my own weight-loss journey:

"I'll get to my ideal weight of 140 pounds in three months".

Additionally, you can create an affirmation based on your idealized self, such as "I am the best salesperson for the month of December."

Advantages of sending a letter of affirmation to oneself

I believe that we frequently fail to seek within for drive and strength. We frequently look outside of ourselves for direction, which is OK, but there are instances when we may use what we already have to achieve where we want to go. We can access or manipulate our sub consciousness to our own advantage to access our intuition and higher selves. You can strengthen your connection to this inner direction by saying daily affirmations or, in this example, penning an affirmation to yourself.

When you begin using affirmations, something within of you changes. Affirmations take different amounts of time to work, but over time, you can anticipate becoming:

- More driven

- More self-assured

- Feeling better about oneself

- Reach milestones you never imagined possible

- Rather than being affected (sometimes negatively), influence others

Applications for affirmation letters

It totally depends on your circumstances and your goals how you compose an affirmation letter to yourself. One of the following few possibilities exists:

1. Writing a letter to oneself to remind yourself of all your wonderful traits and how unique you are is a kind of self-care or self-love.

2. When you want to ask your higher self for advice. In this circumstance, I would find a quiet place to sit and reflect on the problem at hand. Give yourself some time to reflect before beginning to write anything that comes to mind without thinking about using good grammar. Follow your gut instinct.

3. You want to manifest something, such as a new house, success on a test or quiz, or something for

someone. Write your message as if the thing you're attempting to manifest is already a reality. When you're finished, spend a few minutes every day thinking back on what you wrote and feeling like you've already accomplished it.

What should I write in my letter of affirmation?

First, let's take care of a very crucial matter. You are not required to write with flawless English or in the style of a Pulitzer Prize winner. Make it personal and distinctive to you as this is a letter to oneself rather than an exam.

Give yourself no reason not to do it since nobody will judge you for it. The statement "I can't write properly" is not a good excuse and, in fact, should be disregarded because it is a self-limiting belief. All you have to do to write an affirmation letter is make sure you include phrases that are uplifting, positive, and that make you feel good about yourself. Using words that speak to you and that you believe in is crucial in this situation, just as it is when writing affirmations.

Simple instructions for drafting a letter of affirmation to yourself

Now comes the enjoyable part—putting pen to paper. I do, in fact, mean a real pen and paper. In contrast to typing on my phone, I find that writing is more therapeutic and feels more like a real action. It's beneficial to occasionally disconnect from electronics and spend some time by yourself. Once more, I want to emphasize that you should focus on making your affirmation letter unique to you and not spend too much time worrying about grammar, spelling, or organization. Don't overthink the process and refrain from asking, "Oh how am I expected to achieve all that?" Just be yourself, write in the now (not the past or the future), and be yourself. These kinds of inquiries are not pertinent at this time. Embrace the procedure.

Step 1 is to warmly greet oneself.

Use loving and affectionate phrases to greet yourself, just as you would with a loved one, member of your family, or your children. While some might choose something more contemporary like "Hey Boo," I always choose the traditional "Dearest Allyson."

Step 2: Boost your confidence.

Even though you may be going through a difficult moment right now, you know that you did well and made yourself proud. Write encouraging phrases that remind you of your accomplishments and to keep up the excellent work in this situation.

An illustration would be as follows: "My dear Allyson, you are so wonderful with your kids. Due to a death in your family, this time has been difficult, but you have shown incredible strength to keep everyone together. You are the family's rock.

Step 3: Make a commitment to yourself.

I like to make a commitment to myself at the end of my affirmation letters that typically has to do with how I'm doing with growing and appreciating myself. I take this chance to pledge myself that I will take self-love seriously and put it into practice on a regular basis. An illustration would be as follows:

"Despite any flaws I may have, I will always have unconditional love for myself since I am continually working to improve my life. This also applies to my family and close friends. Even when others use harsh language, I don't take it personally since I know better.

How to write a letter of affirmation to yourself

A few more pointers on writing an affirmation to yourself are what I'd like to leave you with.

• Allocate time for this activity. There shouldn't be a sense of urgency or time restriction.

• Locate a nice and quiet area. I enjoy turning down the lights and playing soft music. Avoiding interruptions is crucial when writing.

• I also enjoy sipping on my favorite beverage while doing this, preferably without alcohol.

• Visualize what you want in your mind's eye and write it down as simply as possible.

• Read aloud while you compose.

• From time to time, especially during trying times, read your letter again.

Meditation for Cancer Patients

Numerous cancer treatment facilities now provide meditation as a "alternative" therapy since it may have several advantages for cancer patients. Among other symptoms, potential advantages include a decrease in anxiety and depression, less stress, more energy, and a reduction in chronic pain. There are also not many hazards at the same time. Anyone can start at any time, unlike many alternative therapies for managing cancer symptoms.

How Does Meditation Work?

The most straightforward definition of meditation is the practice of finding a peaceful place to sit, letting go of concerns about the past and the future, and concentrating on the here and now. The aim of mindfulness meditation is to calm your mind and allow you to be fully present in the moment, free from intrusive ideas. Focusing on a sense, such as your breathing, during meditation may involve only observing it without judgment or analysis. To enter a meditative state, some people repeat a phrase or a mantra; while others let their minds wander. Meditation is most frequently practiced while sitting still, however it can also be done while engaging in mild activities (for example, walking meditation). Self-directed or guided meditations are both possible.

Benefits

There are numerous advantages of meditation for overall health and wellbeing. It has been demonstrated to lower blood pressure, alleviate tension in the muscles, and elevate mood. By focusing their thoughts and blocking out worries about the future and regrets about the past, meditation has been shown to assist many people emotionally regain a sense of serenity. But those with cancer may also benefit specifically from meditation. A few of these are:

Anxiety and depression

One study discovered that mindfulness-based cognitive treatment for cancer patients reduced their depressive symptoms. These effects persisted three months later, in contrast to some alternative therapies that only offer cancer patients temporary relief.

Stress

According to numerous researches, meditation greatly reduces cancer patients' perceptions of stress. This advantage may extend beyond the general feeling of wellbeing that results from lower stress and instead support a stronger immune system. Chemicals known as stress hormones, which are released in our bodies in response to stress, may influence survival as well as how effectively someone responds to cancer treatment. According to one study, meditation helped persons with breast and prostate cancer lower their stress hormone levels, and the benefits persisted a year later. Th1 cytokines are inflammatory substances produced by the body that may influence how we react to cancer and how we recover from cancer. Meditation has been shown to reduce these levels.

Continual Pain

A typical and often annoying symptom of cancer is chronic pain. The root cause could be the cancer itself, its treatments, or secondary factors. Regardless of the etiology, almost 90% of persons with lung cancer are thought to have some level of pain. Meditation seems to alleviate this pain and may reduce the amount of painkillers required to regulate pain.

Sleep Issues

For persons with cancer, sleep problems are a typical issue. According to studies, meditation leads to better sleep quality and decreased insomnia.

Cognitive Ability

Cognitive dysfunction is prevalent and can be brought on by either the cancer itself or by cancer therapies like chemotherapy (chemo brain). According to at least one study, meditation helps cancer patients' cognitive functioning.

Fatigue

One of the most irritating side effects of cancer and cancer treatment is cancer fatigue. According to studies, meditation may help cancer patients feel more energized and less worn out.

Cautions

For persons with cancer, meditation is typically a fairly safe activity. Nevertheless, some people may experience anxiety and others may experience disorientation while meditating. It's crucial to emphasize that this is for those who use meditation in addition to or as part of an integrative treatment plan for cancer, such as chemotherapy and other traditional cancer treatments. There is currently no proof that meditation or any other therapy may treat cancer itself, and utilizing these therapies in place of conventional cancer treatments has been associated with a significantly increased risk of death for cancer patients.

What to Do First

Today, a number of sizable cancer centers provide classes in meditation to get you started. Whether not, ask your oncologist if she is aware of any classes or practitioners who could help you start meditating in your region. You can learn and practice meditation at home, which is a good thing. Online resources for learning how to meditate, as well as movies that can help with meditation (such guided imagery), are available for free, around-the-clock.

Cancer-related myths

On the internet, there are unsettling claims that commonplace items and products, including plastic and deodorant, might cause cancer. In addition to being false, many of these misconceptions could make you worry unduly about your families and your own health.

Take a peek at the truth behind these widespread beliefs before you start to worry.

Myth: Deodorants or antiperspirants can lead to breast cancer.

Factual statement: There is insufficient proof to link the usage of underarm deodorants or antiperspirants with breast cancer.

According to some accounts, these products may include dangerous ingredients including aluminum compounds and parabens that can enter the body through cuts from shaving or can be absorbed through the skin. The topic of whether these products cause breast cancer is still open, and no conclusive clinical studies have yet provided a response. But current research indicates that these products do not appear to be carcinogenic. Choose deodorant or antiperspirant that doesn't include ingredients that bother you if you're still afraid that they may raise your chance of cancer.

Myth: Heating food in plastic wraps and containers causes the release of carcinogens.

Factual statement: Plastic wraps and containers with microwave safety labels are safe to use. Some data suggests that plastic containers not suited for microwave use may melt and possibly leak toxins into your food. Never microwave plastic containers like margarine tubs, takeaway containers, or whipped topping bowls since they were not made for the microwave. Verify that every container you use in the microwave has the designation "microwave safe" on the label.

Myth: Sugar shouldn't be consumed by cancer patients because it can hasten the disease's progression.

Factual statement: The link between dietary sugar and cancer need further research, it is a fact. Every cell type, including cancer cells, depends on glucose (blood sugar) for energy. However, feeding cancer cells more sugar doesn't cause them to multiply more quickly. Similarly, cancer cells don't develop more slowly when their access to sugar is cut off. This misperception may have its roots in an incorrect understanding of positron emission tomography (PET) scans, which employ a small quantity of radioactive tracer, frequently in the form of glucose. All of the tissues in your body take up some of this tracer, but the more energetic tissues, such as cancer cells, take up more of it. Some have come to the conclusion that cancer cells grow more quickly on sugar for this reason. However, this is untrue. There is some evidence to suggest that excessive sugar consumption raises the chance of developing various malignancies, particularly esophageal cancer. Consuming excessive amounts of sugar can raise weight, increase the risk of obesity and diabetes, and even increase the chance of cancer.

Myth: Cancer spreads easily.

Factual statement: You shouldn't avoid those who have cancer. It escapes your grasp. Spending time and touching someone who has cancer is acceptable. Your assistance could not possibly be more crucial. Even while viruses can spread easily, cancer can also emerge from infectious viruses on occasion. Viruses that have been known to cause cancer include:

• The sexually transmitted disease known as the human papillomavirus (HPV), which can lead to cancers other than cervical cancer.

• Hepatitis B or C, viruses that can lead to liver cancer and are spread through sex or the use of infected IV needles.

Discuss vaccinations and other methods of virus defense with your doctor.

Chapter 4

True healing from nutrients- the metabolic approach

Food is ingested and utilized by the body through the process of nutrition for tissue repair, growth, and maintenance. A healthy diet is essential for optimum health. A healthy diet consists of foods and beverages that supply the body with essential elements (vitamins, minerals, protein, carbs, fat, and water). Cancer patients will be helped to maintain a healthy body weight, retain their strength, and lessen side effects both before and after treatment by eating primarily plant-based meals and engaging in regular exercise. Nutritional adverse effects might result from cancer and cancer therapy. When tumors affect the head, neck, esophagus, stomach, intestines, pancreas, or liver, nutrition issues are likely to occur. The side effects of cancer therapies make it challenging for many people to eat healthfully. The following cancer therapies have an impact on nutrition:

- Chemotherapy.

- Hormone treatment.

- Radiation treatment.

- Surgery.

- Immunotherapy.

- A transplant of stem cells.

Malnutrition can result from cancer and its therapies.

Taste, smell, appetite, and the capacity to consume enough food or absorb nutrients from food can all be impacted by cancer and cancer therapies. Malnutrition, a disorder brought on by a lack of essential nutrients, may result from this. Malnutrition may be more likely in people who abuse alcohol and are obese. A patient who is malnourished may become weak, exhausted, and unable to fend off an infection or complete cancer therapy. Malnutrition can therefore worsen the patient's quality of life and perhaps endanger their life. The progression or spread of the cancer may exacerbate malnutrition. Protein and calories must be consumed in the proper proportions to promote healing, fight illness, and provide adequate energy.

Loss of appetite or desire to eat is a symptom of anorexia. It is a typical symptom among cancer patients. If the cancer develops or spreads, anorexia may develop early in the illness or later. When given a cancer diagnosis, some people already struggle with anorexia. Anorexia affects the majority of cancer patients with advanced disease. The most frequent reason for malnutrition in cancer patients is anorexia.

Weaknesses, weight loss, as well as the loss of fat and muscle, are symptoms of cachexia. Patients with malignancies that interfere with eating and digesting frequently experience it. Cancer patients who are eating well but are not retaining fat and muscle due to tumor growth may experience it.

Some tumors alter how the body utilizes particular nutrients. Tumors in the stomach, intestines, head and neck may alter how the body uses protein, carbs, and fat. Even though a patient may appear to be eating enough, the body may not be able to fully absorb the nutrients from the meal.

Anorexia and cachexia can coexist in cancer patients.

Nutritional Impacts of Cancer Treatment

Hormone therapy and chemotherapy

The entire body is affected by chemotherapy on the cells. Chemotherapy uses medications to either kill cancer cells or prevent them from proliferating in order to stop the growth of cancer cells. It is also possible to kill healthy cells that would ordinarily proliferate and expand swiftly. These include the digestive tract and oral cells. In hormone therapy, hormones are added, blocked, or removed. Certain cancers may be treated with it to stop or reduce their growth. Weight gain may result from some hormone therapy treatments. Chemotherapy side effects might make it difficult to consume and digest food. Each chemotherapy medicine may have different adverse effects when administered in combination with another treatment, or when two drugs have the same side effect, the side effect may be more severe.

Common negative effects include:

• Appetite loss.

• Nausea.

• Vomiting.

• Mouth ache.

• Mouth- or throat-related sores.

• Modifications to food flavor.

- Difficulty swallowing

- After consuming a tiny amount of food, feeling full.

- Constipation.

- Diarrhea.

Patients who get hormone therapy might need to make dietary adjustments to avoid gaining weight.

Radiation treatment

In the treatment region, radiation therapy kills both cancerous and healthy cells. Among the following factors, they determine how serious the adverse effects are:

- The body portion that is being treated.

- The overall radiation dose and the method of delivery

Nutritional issues can result from the negative effects of radiation therapy on any part of the digestive system. The majority of the adverse effects appears two to three weeks into radiation therapy and disappears a few weeks later. Some side effects may last for months or even years.

Some of the most frequent negative effects include the following:

• For radiation therapy to the head, neck, or brain

•Appetite loss.

• Nausea.

•Vomiting.

•Thick or dry mouth saliva. A dry mouth may be treated with medication.

•Sore gums and mouth.

•A change in the flavor of the dish.

• Swallowing issues.

•Swallowing discomfort

•The mouth not being able to fully open.

Chest radiation therapy

•Appetite loss.

•Nausea.

•Vomiting.

•Swallowing issues.

•Swallowing discomfort

•Breathing or choking issues brought on by alterations in the upper esophagus.

Radiation treatment of the pelvis, rectum, or abdomen

•Nausea.

•Vomiting.

•Stomach obstruction

•Colitis.

•Diarrhea.

Additionally, fatigue brought on by radiation therapy may result in a loss of appetite.

Surgery

To mend wounds, fight infection, and recuperate from surgery, the body requires additional energy and nutrition. Before surgery, the patient's nutrition may be inadequate, which could result in complications including infection or poor healing. Before surgery, nutrition care may start for these individuals. Surgery is typically used to treat cancer patients. Surgery that removes all or a portion of a patient's organs may impair their capacity to consume and process food.

Surgery-related dietary issues include the following:

• Appetite loss.

• Difficulty chewing

• Difficulty swallowing

• Satiation after consuming a tiny amount of food.

Immunotherapy

Depending on the immunotherapy medicine used and the patient, different adverse effects may be experienced.

The following dietary issues are frequent:

• Tiredness.

• Fever.

• Nausea.

• Vomiting.

• Diarrhea.

Stem Cell Replacement

Before or after a stem cell transplant, chemotherapy, radiation therapy, and other medications may have adverse effects that prevent the patient from regularly eating and digesting food.

These are some typical negative effects:

• Sore throats and mouths.

• Diarrhea.

A stem cell transplant recipient's risk of infection is very great. The quantity of white blood cells that fight infection is decreased by chemotherapy or radiation therapy administered prior to the transplant. It's crucial that these patients understand proper food handling techniques and steer clear of potentially infectious foods. Patients are susceptible to developing acute or chronic graft-versus-host disease following a stem cell transplant (GVHD). GVHD can alter a patient's capacity to eat and absorb nutrients from meals by affecting the liver or digestive system.

Nutritional Evaluation in Cancer Treatment

In order to reduce the danger of inadequate nutrition, screening is done to look for health issues. This can assist in determining whether nutrition therapy is required and whether the patient is likely to become malnourished.

The medical staff might inquire about the following:

• Weight shifts throughout the last 12 months.

• Changes in the type and quantity of food consumed.

• Issues that have interfered with eating, such as pain, nausea, vomiting, diarrhea, constipation, mouth sores, dry mouth, or loss of appetite.

• The capacity to move about and perform other daily tasks (dressing, getting into or out of a bed or chair, taking a bath or shower, and using the toilet).

A physical examination is performed to examine the body for general health and disease symptoms. The patient is examined for indicators of weight loss, fat loss, muscle loss, and fluid accumulation in the body. The patient's nutrition is enhanced by counseling and dietary modifications. Patients and their family can receive advice from a qualified dietician on how to enhance the patient's nutrition. Based on the patient's dietary and nutritional requirements, the registered dietitian provides care. Dietary modifications are designed to assist lessen the effects of cancer and cancer therapy. The types and quantity of food consumed, the frequency of meals, and the manner in which meals are consumed may all alter (for example, at a certain temperature or taken with a straw).

During cancer treatment and recovery, a registered dietician collaborates with other members of the healthcare team to monitor the patient's nutritional status. The medical staff may also consist of the following individuals in addition to the dietitian:

• Physician.

• Nurse.

• A social worker

• Psychologist.

Giving patients with advanced cancer the highest quality of life, while managing uncomfortable symptoms is the main aim of nutrition treatment. Patients with advanced cancer may receive palliative care alone, palliative care along with anticancer therapy or hospice care. Each patient will have distinct nutritional objectives. If a certain course of treatment is not benefiting the patient, it may be discontinued.

Nutritional goals may become less aggressive as the focus of care shifts from cancer therapy to hospice or end-of-life care, and a move to care designed to keep the patient as comfortable as possible.

Therapy for Symptoms

Changes can be made to assist the patient in obtaining the nutrients they require when cancer-related side effects or cancer therapy disrupt normal eating. It's crucial to consume foods that are high in calories, protein, vitamins, and minerals. Meals should be prepared to suit the patient's dietary preferences and needs. The symptoms induced by cancer and its treatments, as well as methods for treating or managing them, are listed here.

Anorexia

Cancer patients with anorexia (lack of appetite or desire to eat) may benefit from the following:

• Consume foods that are high in calories and protein. The following foods are high in protein:

•Beans.

•Chicken.

•Fish.

•Meat.

•Yogurt.

•Eggs.

Increase the protein and caloric content of food by adding protein-fortified milk, for example.

• When your appetite is the greatest, start your meal with high-protein items.

• Drink little to no liquids while eating.

•If you don't feel like eating solid things, sip on milkshakes, smoothies, juices, or soups.

• Consume savory dishes.

• Examine new dishes and cuisines.

• Examine nutrient-dense beverages made in blenders.

• Frequently during the day, eat modest meals and wholesome snacks.

• When you feel good and are rested, eat larger meals.

• Whether it's at breakfast, lunch, or supper, eat the largest meal you can when you're most hungry.

• Prepare little quantities of your favorite foods and store them so they are available when you are hungry.

• Keep yourself as active as you can to maintain a healthy appetite.

•To ease symptoms and aftertastes, brush your teeth and swish water around your mouth.

• Consult a certified dietitian or your doctor if you have nausea, vomiting, or changes in the flavor or odor of your food.

To ensure that you receive enough nutrients each day, tube feedings may be required if these dietary adjustments are ineffective in treating anorexia.

Nausea

Cancer patients who experience nausea may find the following helpful:

• Pick foods that you enjoy. Never make yourself consume something that makes you feel ill. Avoid associating your favorite meals with being unwell by avoiding them.

• Opt for bland, soft, and simple-to-digest foods over filling meals.

• Snack on dry foods all day long, such as toast, bread sticks, or crackers.

• Consume simple, stomach-friendly foods like white bread, plain yogurt, and clear soup.

•If you get morning sickness, eat dry toast or crackers before getting out of bed.

• Consume food and beverages at room temperature (not too hot or too cold).

• Drink beverages gradually throughout the day.

• If your mouth tastes terrible, suck on firm candies like peppermints or lemon drops.

• Steer clear of odor-intensive foods and beverages.

• Rather than 3 substantial meals a day, eat 5 or 6 smaller ones.

• To avoid feeling full or bloated during meals, drink very little liquid.

• Avoid skipping meals or snacks. Having an empty stomach could make you feel sicker.

• After eating and before bed, rinse your mouth.

• Avoid eating in a warm or smelly place when you're cooking. Maintain a comfortable temperature and adequate ventilation in the living area.

• One hour after eating, stand up or lie down with your head up.

• Consider when you should eat and drink.

• Unwind prior to every cancer therapy.

• Put on comfortable, loose-fitting clothing.

• Note the times and causes of your nausea.

• Discuss utilizing nausea medications with your doctor.

Vomiting

Cancer patients who experience nausea may find the following helpful:

• Refrain from eating or drinking anything until the nausea passes.

• After vomiting stops, sip small amounts of clear liquids.

• Once you can drink clear liquids without throwing up, start consuming stomach-friendly drinks like milkshakes or strained soups.

• Rather than 3 substantial meals a day, eat 5 or 6 smaller ones.

• After vomiting, sit erect and lean forward.

• Request medication for vomiting management or prevention from your doctor.

Dry mouth

Dry mouth caused by cancer treatment of patients may be relieved by the following:

• Consume foods that are simple to digest.

• Use salad dressing, sauce, or gravy to moisten food.

• Consume highly sweet or tangy meals and beverages, such lemonade, to promote salivation.

• Suck on hard candies, ice pops, or ice chips, or chew gum.

• Drink water all day long.

• Avoid consuming any alcohol, including wine and beer.

• Avoid meals that may irritate your mouth (such as spicy, sour, salty, hard, or crunchy foods).

• Use lip balm to keep your lips moisturized.

• Rinse your mouth once or twice every hour. Avoid using alcohol based mouthwash.

• Abstain from cigarette use and limit exposure to secondhand smoke.

• Discuss utilizing artificial saliva or comparable items to coat, safeguard, and moisten your mouth and throat with your doctor or dentist.

Oral sores

The following can assist people with mouth sores:

• Consume soft, simple-to-chew foods like custards, milkshakes, and scrambled eggs.

• Cook food until it is tender and soft.

• Chop food into bite-sized pieces. To smooth food, use a blender or food processor.

• To numb and calm your mouth, take a sip of ice chips.

• Consume food at room temperature or cold. You can burn your mouth eating hot food.

• Use a straw to drink in order to get liquid past the sore spots in your mouth.

• To make it simpler to chew your food, use a small spoon to assist you take smaller bits.

Steer clear of the following:

•Oranges, lemons, and limes are examples of citrus fruits.

•Spicy dishes.

•Ketchup with tomatoes.

•Salty dishes.

•Raw produce.

•food that are sour and crunchy.

•Drinks that contain alcohol

• Abstain from tobacco use.

•Schedule an appointment with a dentist at least two weeks before beginning immunotherapy, chemo, or radiation treatment for the head and neck.

•Look for sores, white patches, or puffy and red areas in your mouth every day.

• Mouthwash three to four times per day. For a mouthwash, combine 1 cup warm water, 1/8 teaspoon salt, and 1/4 teaspoon baking soda. Avoid using mouthwash with alcohol in it.

• Avoid using toothpicks or any other pointed things.

Changes in Tastes

The following could benefit cancer patients who experience changes in taste:

• Replace red meat with poultry, fish, eggs, and cheese.

• Season food with sauces and spices (marinate foods).

• Pair meat with a sweet food, such applesauce, jam, or cranberry sauce.

• Try sour foods and beverages.

• If your mouth is leaving you with a metallic or bitter taste, try sugar-free lemon drops, gum, or mints.

• If food tastes metallic, use plastic utensils and avoid drinking straight from metal containers.

• If you are not sick, try to eat some of your favorite meals. When you're feeling your best, try new meals.

• A vegetarian or Chinese cookbook may contain non-meat, high-protein meals.

•If food tastes bland but not unpleasant, chew it for a longer period of time to allow greater contact with taste buds.

• If odors disturb you, cook outside or use a fan in the kitchen while cooking.

•Keep foods and beverages covered.

• Clean your mouth and brush your teeth. Checkups should be done at the dentist.

Throat ache and difficulty swallowing

Cancer patients who experience a painful throat or difficulty swallowing may benefit from the following:

• Consume soft, simple-to-chew, and simple-to-swallow foods like milkshakes, scrambled eggs, oatmeal, or other prepared cereals.

• Consume calorie- and protein-dense foods and beverages.

• Add gravy, sauces, broth, or yogurt to moisten dishes.

Avoid the following foods and beverages that can irritate or burn your throat:

•Warm foods and beverages.

•Spicy dishes.

• Foods and juices that is strong in acid.

•Meal that is sour or crunchy.

•Drinks that contain alcohol

• Cook food until it is tender and soft.

• Chop food into bite-sized pieces. To smooth food, use a blender or food processor.

• Sip via a straw.

• Rather than 3 substantial meals a day, eat 5 or 6 smaller ones.

• When you eat or drink, sit upright with your head bowed slightly forward. After eating, maintain this position for at least 30 minutes.

• Do not use tobacco.

If you are unable to eat enough to maintain your strength, speak to your doctor about tube feedings.

Intolerance to lactose

Patients who experience lactose intolerance symptoms may benefit from the following:

• Use milk products that are lactose-free or low-lactose. The majority of grocery stores sell foods with the labels "lactose free" or "reduced lactose," including milk and ice cream.

• Opt for low-lactose dairy products like yogurt and hard cheeses (like cheddar).

• Try soy or rice-based goods (such as soy and rice milk and frozen desserts). There is no lactose in these items.

• Only steer clear of the dairy products that cause you issues. If you can, consume tiny amounts of dairy products like milk, yogurt, or cheese.

• Try consuming calcium-enriched nondairy beverages and meals.

• Consume vegetables high in calcium, like broccoli and leafy greens.

• Take lactase supplements if you consume dairy products. Lactose is broken down by lactase to make it simpler to digest.

• Make your own lactose-free or low-lactose foods.

Gaining Weight

Cancer sufferers may find the following helpful in preventing weight gain:

• Fill up on fresh fruit and vegetables.

• Consume high-fiber foods, such as whole-grain pasta, breads, and cereals.

• Opt for lean meats like lean beef, pork that has been fat-trimmed, and poultry (like chicken or turkcy) without skin.

• Opt for low-fat dairy products.

• Eat fewer fats (eat only small amounts of butter, mayonnaise, desserts, and fried foods).

• Use low-fat cooking techniques including broiling, steaming, grilling, or roasting.

•Consume less salt.

• Fill up on meals you like to feel content.

• Just eat when you're hungry. If you eat as a result of stress, fear, or depression, think about seeking counseling or medication. Find activities you like to do if you eat because you're bored.

• At meals, consume less calories.

• Everyday exercise.

• Consult your doctor before beginning a weight-loss diet.

Nutritional Supports

When feasible, it is recommended to eat by mouth. A patient's ability to swallow enough food may be compromised if they have cancer or cancer treatment-related issues. Nutrition therapy also involves nutritional supplement drinks, enteral and parenteral nutrition support, advice from a dietician, and dietary adjustments. Cancer patients who consume nutritional supplement beverages can acquire the nutrients they require. Energy, protein, fat, carbs, fiber, vitamins, and minerals are all provided by them. They shouldn't be the only source of nutrients for the sufferer. If a patient is unable to consume the recommended number of calories and nutrients orally, they may be fed using one of the following methods:

Enteral nutrition

The administration of nutrients via a tube placed in the intestines or stomach. While nutrition support can enhance a patient's quality of life while receiving cancer treatment, there are some drawbacks that should be taken into account before using it. The patient and medical staff should talk about the advantages and disadvantages of each method of nutrition support.

Through a tube inserted into the stomach or small intestine, enteral feeding provides the patient with nutrients in liquid form (formula). It is possible to utilize the subsequent kinds of feeding tubes:

• The stomach or small intestine is reached by inserting a nasogastric tube via the nose and down the throat. When enteral nourishment is only required for a few weeks, this is employed.

• Through an incision created on the exterior of the abdomen, a gastrostomy tube is placed into the stomach or a jejunostomy tube is placed into the small intestine. This is typically used for patients who cannot utilize a tube in their nose or throat or for long-term enteral feeding.

Based on the patient's unique demands, the type of formula is chosen. There are formulae available for those with specific dietary requirements or medical disorders like diabetes.

Intravenous Nutrition

When the patient is unable to consume food orally or by enteral feeding, parenteral nutrition is employed. With parenteral feeding, food is not broken down in the stomach or intestines. Through a catheter placed in a vein, nutrients are administered to the patient straight into the blood. These nutrients include vitamins, minerals, lipids, and proteins. Under the skin, a central venous access catheter is inserted into a sizable vein in the upper chest. An orthopedic surgeon inserts the catheter. Long-term parenteral nutrition is provided using this kind of catheter.

A central venous catheter is a small, flexible tube that is threaded into the superior vena cava, a significant vein above the right side of the heart, usually below the right collarbone. Injectable fluids, blood transfusions, chemotherapy, and other medications are administered through it. Blood samples can also be drawn using the catheter. It helps prevent the need for recurrent needle sticks and may remain in place for weeks or months.

A tiny, bendable tube called a peripheral venous catheter is placed into a vein. A vein in the arm is used to insert a peripheral venous catheter. Medical professionals with the appropriate training install a peripheral venous catheter. For patients without a central venous access catheter, this kind of catheter is typically utilized for intermittent parenteral nutrition. It is typically put into the back of the hand or the bottom portion of the arm. Injectable fluids, blood transfusions, chemotherapy, and other medications are administered through it. The patient is checked often for infection or bleeding at the point where the catheter enters the body.

Drugs for Treating Appetite Loss and Weight Loss

Early treatment of cancer symptoms and side effects that impair eating and result in weight loss is crucial. Cancer and its treatment can have a negative impact on weight loss, but this can be mitigated with both nutrition therapy and medication.

Prednisone and megestrol, two drugs that increase appetite and promote weight gain, may be used to treat anorexia and weight loss. According to studies, these medications' effects may be short-lived or nonexistent. Combination therapy may be more effective than single-medicament therapy. Patients who take many medications at once may experience more negative effects.

Dietary Needs at the End of Life

The objectives of nutrition treatment for patients who are nearing the end of their lives are more concerned with symptom relief than with consuming enough nutrients.

The following list of typical signs of end-of-life conditions:

•Anorexia (loss of appetite).

• Mouth ache.

• Issues with swallowing.

• Nausea.

• Vomiting.

Thicker liquids may be simpler for patients who have trouble swallowing than thinner ones. Patients may only want a small amount of food and frequently do not feel really hungry. In the latter days of life, oral care, ice chips, and water sips can quench your thirst. Understanding the patient's changing nutritional needs requires effective communication with the medical team. The right to make informed decisions extends to those who are caring for cancer patients. The patient's decisions may be influenced by their religious and cultural inclinations. When making decisions, the healthcare staff may consult with the patient's religious and cultural leaders. The advantages and drawbacks of providing nutrition support for patients towards the end of life might be discussed between the medical team and a trained dietician. There are typically more negative effects than positive ones.

The following are some dangers of feeding supplementation for the terminally ill:

• Sepsis with parenteral feeding (bacteria or their toxins in the blood or tissues).

• Aspiration caused by enteral feeding, which is the unintentional inhalation of food or liquid into the lungs.

• Skin breakdown and sores at the location of the enteral feeding tube.

• Diarrhea when receiving nourishment via parenteral and enteral routes.

• Issues with enteral and parenteral feeding due to fluid overload (a condition in which there is too much fluid in the blood).

Food Trends and Cancer

Special diets may be tried by cancer patients to improve the effectiveness of their treatments, reduce unwanted effects from treatments, or even to treat the cancer itself. There is, however, no proof that the majority of these special diets are effective.

Vegan or vegetarian food

It is unknown if adopting a vegetarian or vegan diet can improve the patient's prognosis or lessen the negative effects of cancer treatment. There is no proof that a patient who already consumes a vegetarian or vegan diet needs to change their diet.

Macrobiotic diet

A macrobiotic diet consists of a lot of plant-based carbohydrates and little fat. No research has indicated that this diet will benefit people with cancer.

ketogenic diet

A ketogenic diet restricts carbs while elevating fat consumption. Dietary restrictions are used to limit the amount of glucose (sugar) the tumor cells may absorb and use for growth and reproduction. Because precise proportions of lipids, carbohydrates, and proteins must be consumed, the diet is challenging to follow. But the diet is secure. Glioblastoma patients are being enrolled in several clinical trials to determine whether a ketogenic diet has an impact on the tumor activity of this disease. Glioblastoma patients who wish to begin a ketogenic diet should consult their physician and a trained dietitian. How the diet will impact the tumor or its symptoms, though, is not yet known. In a similar vein, the ketogenic diet was found to be both safe and acceptable in a research comparing it to a high-fiber, low-fat diet in women with endometrial or ovarian cancer. The effects of the ketogenic diet on ovarian or endometrial cancers or their signs and symptoms are unknown.

Supplemental nutrition may be used by some cancer patients. A product added to the diet is referred to as a dietary supplement. It typically contains one or more dietary components and is taken by mouth.

Supplements for the diet can help cancer patients manage their symptoms or treat their disease.

Vitamin C

The body need trace amounts of vitamin C to function and maintain health. It assists with infection control, wound healing, and tissue health. Veggies and fruits contain vitamin C. Additionally, it is available as a dietary supplement.

Probiotics

Live bacteria called probiotics are used as dietary supplements to support healthy digestion and bowel function. They might also promote the health of the digestive system. According to studies, eating probiotics during chemotherapy and radiation therapy can lessen the risk of developing diarrhea as a side effect. Patients who receive radiation treatment to the abdomen can rely on this. Probiotics may be beneficial for cancer patients receiving chemotherapy or abdominal radiation therapy that is known to produce diarrhea. Similar research is being done on the advantages of probiotics for cancer patients receiving immunotherapy.

Melatonin

The pineal gland produces a hormone called melatonin (tiny organ near the center of the brain). The body's sleep cycle is regulated by melatonin. Additionally, it can be created in a lab and used as a dietary supplement. A number of modest studies have suggested that it might be beneficial to combine melatonin supplements with chemotherapy and/or radiation therapy for the treatment of solid tumors. It might lessen adverse effects from medication. There don't seem to be any negative consequences of melatonin.

Fating glutamine

An amino acid called oral glutamine is being investigated for the treatment of diarrhea and mucositis, an inflammation of the digestive tract's lining that frequently manifests as mouth sores, brought on by chemotherapy or radiation therapy. Glutamate taken orally may lessen the severity of or aid to avoid mucositis. Oral glutamine may be helpful for cancer patients getting radiation therapy to the abdomen. Glutamate taken orally may lessen the severity of diarrhea. The patients' ability to carry out their treatment plan can be aided by this.

Tea and Breakfast plan for Cancer patients

Patients receiving chemotherapy have discovered that specific breakfast foods and types of teas are very beneficial in reducing the impact on their stomachs. The best recommendations are:

Tea with ginger root

Making your own ginger tea is as simple as adding boiling water to ginger root slices and letting them simmer. Ginger has been proved to prevent nausea and vomiting in addition to boosting appetite, which is crucial for cancer patients. Studies have indicated that it aids in the treatment of some cancers, particularly ovarian cancer. This tea is a wonderful choice if you like to buy tea bags that have already been produced because it is made completely of dried ginger root chunks. When choosing a ginger tea, use caution because many products include black or green tea leaves, which are not advised for those receiving some types of chemotherapy.

Tea with peppermint

The well-known antidote for nausea is mint. Drinking it and breathing in its calming aroma can both help people who are experiencing stomach discomfort. Mint is known to benefit people with memory and focus challenges, which are frequent in chemotherapy patients, in addition to easing stomach discomfort. Mint is also an immune system booster.

Milk Thistle Tea

The effectiveness of milk thistle does not lie in its ability to treat nausea; rather, it is known to be a potent stimulant for the liver, which is the organ in charge of eliminating waste and toxins from our blood. As a result, milk thistle will aid in the removal of chemotherapy drugs from our systems once they are no longer required. Additionally, it works well as an anti-inflammatory. One word of caution: consult your doctor before adding milk thistle tea to your cupboard as there are several cancers for which it is explicitly contraindicated.

Valerian root brew

The inability to sleep, one of chemotherapy's more difficult side effects, is combated by valerian. The well-known stress reliever valerian has long been advocated as an effective remedy for insomnia.

Tea with licorice root

Licorice root has a taste that will transport you back to your childhood while also offering you health advantages. It has a reputation for strengthening the immune system and many people think that it can actually help shrink cancer tumors, but before you start drinking it, it's important to talk to your doctor because some studies suggest that it can weaken muscles and suppress the production of hormones that fight stress. If your doctor gives the go-ahead, you can consume it knowing that it is a powerful liver stimulant that will aid in flushing chemotherapy medications from your system once they are no longer required.

Chickpea Pancakes with Almond Butter & Jellyberry Grape Jam

This recipe for wholesome and mouthwatering pancakes will have you flipping. Each pancake is topped with almond butter and Jellyberry grape jam, which is a naturally sweet, home-made jam produced from gluten-free chickpea flour and almond milk. Jellyberry grapes have a naturally sweet, deep, and rich flavor that is comparable to grape jam. They are dark purple, which means they are high in antioxidants that are good for your health. To lower your chance of developing cancer and other diseases, the American Institute for Cancer

Research advises eating at least 312 cups of fruits and vegetables daily. Bright grapes, like the jellyberries in this recipe, help you get one delicious step closer to that goal.

Ingredients

As for the Jam:

- 2 cups halved purple grapes

- Lemon juice, 2 tablespoons

- 1 teaspoon honey

- 1/4 teaspoon cinnamon powder

- A dash of salt for flavor

- 1 tablespoon cornstarch

- 1 tablespoon water

To make the pancakes:

- Chickpea flour, 1 cup

- 2 tablespoons baking powder

- 1/4 teaspoon cinnamon powder

- A dash of salt, or as desired

- 3/4 cup plain almond milk without added sugar

- 1 teaspoon honey

- .5 teaspoons of vanilla extract

- Cooking oil nonstick

- 4 tablespoons of peanut or almond butter

Serves 4. 240 calories, 11 g total fat (1 g saturated fat, 0 g trans-fat), 0 mg of cholesterol, 29 g of carbs, 9 g of protein, 5 g of dietary fiber, 45 mg of sodium, 14 g of sugar, and 3 g of added sugar are all contained in one serving.

Directions

1. Heat a small saucepan to a moderate temperature. Stir in the grapes, honey, cinnamon, salt, and lemon juice. Bring to a low boil, reduce heat, and simmer, covered, stirring periodically, for about 8 minutes, or until grapes soften.

2. Combine cornstarch and water in a small bowl using a whisk. Add to grape mixture and whisk continuously for 1 to 2 minutes, or until thickened. Place aside.

3. In the meantime, combine the chickpea flour, baking soda, cinnamon, and salt in a medium basin. Almond

milk, honey, and vanilla should all be thoroughly blended.

4. Use nonstick cooking spray to coat a 10-inch nonstick skillet, then heat it on medium heat. Pour in 1/3 cup of batter and cook for 2 to 3 minutes, or until the bottom is brown. Should the bottom brown too soon, lower the heat to medium-low. 2 more minutes of cooking follow the flip. Repeat using the remaining batter and frying spray. Between batches, keep the pancakes warm.

5. To assemble, evenly distribute 1 tablespoon of almond butter over each pancake. Add Jellyberry grape jam equally on top.

Notes

There are four 8-inch pancakes from this recipe. You can cook pancakes in any size you like.

Fresh Fruit Oatmeal

With this fresh fruit oatmeal, you can have a great morning. Like all whole grains, rolled oats are a good source of fiber, phytochemicals, vitamins, and minerals. Consuming whole grains has been linked to a lower risk of colorectal cancer, and oatmeal's soluble fiber can also help control blood cholesterol levels. Flaxseed, chopped walnuts, and seasonal fruit give added nutrition and healthy omega-3 fatty acids.

Ingredients

- 1/2 cup rolled old-fashioned oats

- 1 1/4 cups split almond milk

- One tablespoon of ground flaxseed to taste

- 1/2 tsp. of cinnamon

- 1/2 cup pineapple, chopped

- One-fourth cup of sliced strawberries

- 2 tablespoons chopped walnuts, if desired

- Optional 1 teaspoon honey

Yields one serving. 370 calories, 16 g of total fat (1.5 g saturated, 0 g trans), 0 mg of cholesterol, 50 g of carbs, 10 g of protein, 8 g of dietary fiber, 200 mg of sodium, 16 g of sugar, and 0 g of added sugar are all contained in one serving.

Directions

1. Prepare oats in a small pan with 1 cup milk as directed on the packet.

2. Fill the serving basin with oatmeal. Add 1/4 cup milk to the oats (heat milk if preferred). Cinnamon and flaxseed should be added.

3. If preferred, add pineapple, strawberries, walnuts, and honey to the top.

Notes

*An alternate plant-based milk product or low-fat dairy milk can be utilized.

Crepes of chickpeas with a pesto of spinach and mushrooms

Make these crepes quickly for a tasty and light lunch. What's the recipe for these delicate pancakes? They contain besan, a chickpea-based flour (also known as garbanzo bean or gram flour). Besan is rich in protein and fiber because it is made from beans. According to research, diets rich in plant foods, such as beans, can help reduce the chance of developing cancer.

Ingredients

•Chickpea flour, 1 cup

- 2 Tbsp. unrefined olive oil

- 1 tsp. fresh rosemary cut up finely

- 1/4 tsp. salt

- 1 cup of water

- 2 tsp. buttery spread that is soft if using a skillet

Filling:

- 2 tsp. unrefined olive oil

- 1/4 cup red onion, chopped finely

- 1/3 cup of red bell pepper, chopped finely

- 6 oz. thinly sliced cremini mushrooms (about 2 cups)

- One carton of 5-ounce baby spinach

- 2 tbsp. ready pesto

- To taste, add salt and freshly ground black pepper.

1 6-inch crepe is included in each of the 6 servings. Per serving: 170 calories, 10 grams of total fat (1.5 grams of saturated fat, 0 grams of trans fat), 0 mg of cholesterol, 13 grams of carbs, 5 grams of protein, 3 grams of dietary fiber, 630 mg of sodium, 3 grams of sugar, and 0 grams of added sugar.

Directions

1. Whisk 1 cup water, oil, salt, and chickpea flour in a medium bowl until the mixture is smooth. Allow the batter to thicken for 20 to 30 minutes. Stir to break up any clumps before cooking.

2. When making crepes, heat a nonstick pan over medium-high heat until water dripped into the pan begins to bounce and form balls. Hold the pan at a 45-degree angle with one hand. Pour 14 cup batter near the top of the pan while turning the pan to ensure that the batter flows into a 6-7-inch round crepe. Cook for 1-2 minutes, or until crepe is golden on bottom. Flip the crepe using a large spatula, and cook for 30 seconds or until the bottom is faintly brown. Place crepe on a sizable dish. Spread wax paper on each crepe.

3. Crepes should be cooled to room temperature before being filled, then the plate should be covered in plastic wrap. Keep crepes in the refrigerator for up to 24 hours or up to 8 hours at room temperature.

4. Heat oil in a medium skillet over medium-high heat for the filling. For 2 minutes, while stirring, add the onion. Red peppers should be added after the onions have been cooking for 5 minutes while stirring. Add the

mushrooms and simmer for 5 to 6 minutes, stirring regularly, until the mixture appears moist. Add the spinach and toss to wilt the leaves. Cook for 8 minutes, stirring frequently, or until the filling is cooked and most of the moisture has disappeared.

5. If you've made crepes in advance, wrap them in foil and reheat at 250 degrees for 20 minutes. To assemble crepes, combine 2 tbsp. of pesto in a small bowl. hot water. The filling with pesto. Lay a crepe out on a platter. Each crepe should have 16 of the filling spread over the bottom half before being carefully folded over the filling. With the remaining crepes and filling, repeat. Strawberries and some mesclun leaves can be used to decorate the platter, if desired. Serve right away.

Spanish Omelet with Herbs

A delightful brunch classic, this dish is packed with protein, B vitamins, and cancer-preventing phytonutrients. Eggs are a cheap source of protein and have only 70–80 calories per serving. Red onions, fresh spring herbs, and potatoes are all included in this omelet. Allium vegetables including onions, garlic, and chives contain quercetin and allixin, which may help prevent cancer.

Ingredients

- 1 lb. potatoes that have been peeled, diced, or shred

- 2 Tbsp. unrefined olive oil

- 1/2 cup red onion, chopped

- 2 minced garlic cloves

- 4 big, lightly beaten whole eggs

- 2 lightly beaten egg whites

- 2 Tbsp. fresh parsley, cut finely.

- 2 Tbsp. fresh basil and chives each cut fine.

- Salt, as desired

- Fresh herb sprigs as a garnish (optional)

Contains 4 servings (1 omelet per serving). 240 calories, 12 grams of total fat (2.5 grams of saturated fat, 0 grams of trans fat), 185 mg of cholesterol, 23 grams of carbs, 11 grams of protein, 2 grams of dietary fiber, 105 mg of sodium, 2 grams of sugar, and 0 grams of added sugar per serving.

Directions

1.Insert potatoes in a sizable pan. Submerge in water. Cook for 3 minutes uncovered after bringing to a boil. Get rid of the heat. Potatoes should be soft but not mushy after 10 minutes of standing covered. Good drainage

2. Heat oil over medium heat in a deep 10-inch nonstick skillet. Add the onion and garlic. Cook for around 8 minutes, stirring now and again. Add the potatoes and simmer for a further five minutes.

3. Whites and entire eggs should be combined. Add the chives, basil, and parsley. Adding salt is optional. Put mixture in heated skillet and add potatoes. Once the bottom of the omelet is brown, turn down the heat and cook it uncovered for about 10 minutes.

4. Under the toaster oven, brown the top if desired. Use fresh herb sprigs as a garnish. Serve right away.

Pecan and Apricot Bars

These handmade apricot bars will improve your morning and the breakfast of your children. This recipe contains whole grain oats, which are rich in soluble fiber, selenium, and B vitamins, unlike many commercial granola bars. Incorporating whole-grain snacks into your family's diet is a fantastic approach to increase fiber intake for sustained energy and lowered cancer risk. Real dried apricots include vitamin A and potassium, and pecans lend a hearty bite and added protein strength when combined with silken tofu.

Ingredients

• 3 cups oats for rapid cooking

• 1/2 cup chopped pecans

• 3 cups of grain cereal without sugar (cheerios or shredded wheat)

• 2 cups chopped dried apricots

• 1/4 cup whole wheat flour

• 12 oz. Tofu silken, drained

• 1 big egg

• 50 ml of apple sauce

•0.5 cups of canola oil

• 1 cup of honey

• 1/2 tsp. salt

• 1 Tbsp. grated fresh lemon zest

- 1 Tbsp. vanilla essence

- Canola oil spray for cooking

Serves 24 people. 190 calories, 8 g total fat (1 g saturated fat, 0 g trans fat), 10 mg cholesterol, 30 g carbs, 4 g protein, 3 g dietary fiber, 55 mg sodium, 15 g sugar, and 8 g added sugar are all contained in one meal.

Directions

1. Set oven to 350 degrees Fahrenheit.

2. Oats and pecans should be spread out on a sizable (15x10) baking dish. Bake for 8 to 10 minutes, or until aromatic and light brown.

3. Transfer to a sizable mixing bowl and toss in the cereal, apricots, and flour.

4. In a blender, combine the tofu, egg, applesauce, oil, honey, vanilla, and lemon zest until smooth. The tofu mixture should be folded into the middle of the oat mixture after creating a well there. Spray a 9x13 baking dish with cooking spray, and then evenly distribute the mixture inside.

5. Bake for 35 to 40 minutes, or until golden brown and the center is firm. Use a sharp knife to cut the mixture into bars after allowing it cool completely in the dish.

Oats with pumpkin spice overnight

You can prepare a quick grab-and-go breakfast the night before with only five minutes of work, and it will keep you full all morning. These robust oats with pumpkin spice are a powerhouse of fiber, protein, and cancer-preventing polyphenols. Oats and other whole grains can help with weight management, improve digestion, and reduce the risk of colon cancer.

Ingredients

• Half a cup of rolled oats

• 1/2 cup almond milk without added sugar (or any type of milk)

• A third of a cup of plain, low-fat Greek yogurt

• 1 Tbsp. blended flaxseed

• 2 Tbsp. pureed pumpkin

• 1 Tbsp. maple sugar

• 1/2 tsp. vanilla essence

- 1/2 tsp. ground nutmeg

- 1/4 tsp. ginger powder

- 1/4 tsp. crushed nutmeg

- A dash of salt

Yields one serving. 340 calories, 7 g of total fat (1.5 g of saturated fat, 0 g of trans fat), 10 mg of cholesterol, 52 g of carbs, 16 g of protein, 8 g of dietary fiber, 270 mg of sodium, 17 g of sugar, and 12 g of added sugar are all contained in one serving.

Directions

1. In a medium mixing basin, combine all the ingredients and stir well.

2. To a Mason jar with a tight-fitting cover, add.

3. Overnight storage and refrigeration.

Breakfast toast with grilled chard, feta cheese, and eggs

The ideal way to sneak vegetables into your morning is with this bread version. Because they contain carotenoids, dark leafy greens like Swiss chard are among those foods that fight cancer. In lab tests, carotenoids from dark green leafy vegetables have been shown to slow the growth of some cancer cells, including those that cause stomach, lung, and skin cancers.

Ingredients

- One piece of whole-wheat bread

- Two substantial chard leaves, cut

- 1 tsp. olive juice

- 1 tsp. feta

- 1 thinly sliced hard-boiled egg

Produces 1 serving (1). 220 calories, 12 grams of total fat (3 grams of saturated fat, 0 grams of trans fat), 190 mg of cholesterol, 15 grams of carbs, 7 grams of protein, 3 grams of dietary fiber, 250 mg of sodium, 3 grams of sugar, and 0 grams of added sugar per serving.

Directions

1. Griddle bread.

2. Chard should be softened and halved in size while being sautéed in olive oil.

3. Spread it on your toast, and then top it with a hard-boiled egg and feta cheese.

Notes

*You can use kale or spinach in place of chard.

**Chard can be sautéed with a touch of lemon, chopped garlic, or red pepper flakes.

Toast with cottage cheese, cucumber, and tomato

The greatest time to have this toast is during the summer when tomatoes are in season, but if you can't locate any decent tomatoes, you can still enjoy it all year long with just the cucumber. A half-cup of cottage cheese has 14 grams of protein and is a strong source of calcium.

Ingredients

• One piece of whole-wheat bread

• 1/4 cup low-fat cottage cheese

• 4-5 thin slices of cucumber

• 2 to 3 quartered, thin tomato slices

• Black pepper, cracked (to taste)

150 calories, 3 g of total fat (1 g of saturated fat, 0 g of trans fat), 5 mg of cholesterol, 19 g of carbs, 10 g of protein, 3 g of dietary fiber, 310 mg of sodium, 6 g of sugar, and 0 g of added sugar are found in one serving.

Directions

1. Girdle bread

2. On the bread spread cottage cheese

3. Add black pepper, tomatoes and cucumber slice on top

Banana and Chia Seed Toast with Peanut Butter

Bananas have a pleasant flavor that goes well with peanut butter and are a rich source of potassium and fiber. Chia seeds, a whole grain with high antioxidant content, will increase the amount of protein, fiber, and omega-3 fatty acids in your diet when added to food. They have a mild, nutty flavor and go well on toast, sprinkled over yogurt or oatmeal, or blended into drinks.

Ingredients

• One piece of whole-wheat bread

• 1 Tbsp. Almond butter

- Sliced bananas

- 1 tsp. Chia nut (or flaxseed)

Produces 1 serving (1). 11 g total fat (0 g trans-fat, 0 g saturated fat), 0 mg of cholesterol, 34 g of carbs, 9 g of protein, 4 g of dietary fiber, 220 mg of sodium, 12 g of sugar, and 1 g of added sugar are all present in one serving.

Directions

1. Griddle bread.

2. Toast is covered in peanut butter.

3. Chia seeds and banana slices go on top.

Notes

You can substitute flaxseed for the chia seeds and use almond butter in place of peanut butter.

Easy Lasagna for summer

Delicious roasted eggplant, zucchini, and lycopene-rich tomatoes are all packed into this hearty summer lasagna. Whole-wheat noodles include phytochemicals, which are organic plant substances that protect cells from harm that could cause cancer as well as fiber, which fights cancer. This recipe makes plenty for 12 people, making it suitable for batch cooking or feeding a large group.

Ingredients

- Two lengthwise quartered 3 lb. eggplants.

- 6 large zucchini (about 3 lbs.)

- Canola oil spray for cooking

- 15 oz. Low-fat cottage cheese or ricotta (or a combination of both)

- 2 eggs

- A quarter-cup of grated Parmesan cheese

- 1/2 tsp. crushed nutmeg

- 1/2 tsp. powdered garlic

- 4 cups of tomato sauce low in salt

- 1 lb. No-boil whole-wheat lasagna noodles

- Three cups of semi-skim mozzarella cheese

Serves 12 people. 360 calories, 11 g of total fat (5 g saturated fat, 0 g trans fat), 65 mg of cholesterol, 44 g of carbs, 23 g of protein, 9 g of dietary fiber, 400 mg of sodium, 12 g of sugar, and 0 g of added sugar are all contained in one serving.

Directions

1. Set oven to 450 degrees Fahrenheit. A 13 x 9 x 2-inch baking pan should be greased and saved.

2. Slice the zucchini and eggplant into 1/2-inch-thick pieces. The vegetables should be layered on two baking trays and sprayed with cooking spray on both sides. For around 40 minutes, roast.

3. Oven temperature reduced to 375 degrees F.

4. in the meantime, combine the ricotta and/or cottage cheeses, eggs, Parmesan, nutmeg, and garlic powder in a medium bowl.

5. Spread a thin layer of sauce in the bottom of the pan that has been preheated before assembling. Add a layer of pasta on top. Pasta is covered with a third of the ricotta mixture. Over the ricotta, top with a quarter of the mozzarella. Add a third of the roasted vegetables. Once you have 4 layers of pasta and 3 layers of filling, top with 12 cup of tomato sauce and continue assembling as instructed. The leftover mozzarella cheese should then be sprinkled on top of the remaining sauce.

6. Bake the pan for 30 minutes while it is covered with aluminum foil. Remove the top and bake for a further 15 minutes, or until golden and bubbling. 15 minutes should pass before serving.

Apple-Cranberry-Hazelnut Crumble

Nothing beats fruit-forward meals, which offer savory, colorful, and nutritious takes on classic sweets that are frequently stuffed with extra sugars, refined carbohydrates, and saturated fats. Simple crumbles are one way to enjoy desserts with fruit in them. Just combine healthful grains, spices, and nuts for a crunchy baked covering, and then start with seasonal fruits to make a wonderful fruit filling. You may fit more servings of fruits into your day by consuming more nourishing, fruit-forward sweets, which is a good habit for the whole family. Consuming more colored fruits is associated with a decreased risk of cancer, obesity, and heart disease. This recipe is bursting with the deliciousness of seasonal fruit, including cranberries and apples, which are wonderful for your health. It also contains whole-grain flour and oats, which can lower colon cancer risk, improve gut microbial health, and protect your heart. It's a sweet treat you can feel good about as there isn't much extra sugar.

Ingredients

Fruit Compost:

• 10 oz. unsweetened cranberries, either fresh or frozen.

• Sliced and peeled three medium apples

• 1 orange, juice and zest

• 50 g of brown sugar

Granular crumble topping:

• 1 cup oats, old-fashioned

• 1/3 cup whole wheat flour

• 1/3 cup coarsely chopped hazelnuts

• 1 tsp. cinnamon

• 1 tsp. cardamom

• 1/2 tsp. ginger powder

Pinch of salt (optional)

• One-fourth cup vegetable oil

Serves eight. 240 calories, 11 grams of total fat (1.5 grams of saturated fat, 0 grams of trans fat), 0 mg of cholesterol, 35 grams of carbohydrates, 3 grams of protein, 5 grams of dietary fiber, 0 mg of sodium, 19 grams of sugar, and 9 grams of added sugar per serving.

Directions

1. Set the oven to 375°F.

2. Put apples and cranberries in a 9-inch pie plate or baking pan. Blend in brown sugar, orange juice, and zest. Well, toss.

3. Oats, flour, hazelnuts, cinnamon, cardamom, ginger, and salt, if used, are combined in a small bowl. With a fork, stir in the oil to create a crumbly mixture.

4. Cover the cranberry-apple filling with the crumb topping and bake it uncovered, for 45 to 55 minutes, or until it turns golden.

Protein drinks and snacks

The risk of malnutrition can rise due to the impact of cancer and cancer treatments on appetite. Complications may also be more likely if you don't eat enough. Protein smoothies for cancer patients could be a convenient food option that helps with the disease's fight.

When you don't feel like eating, you can still enhance your nutritional intake by drinking protein-rich beverages like milkshakes, smoothies, and blended drinks. High-protein oral nutritional drinks can assist cancer patients maintain their weight and enhance their quality of life. Protein shakes that are already made are readily available at your neighborhood grocery or health food store. These shakes are handy to store in the fridge and may be used as a snack or when you don't feel like eating a full meal.

Sadly, a lot of pre-made protein smoothies might have a lot of added sugar. Try some of the high-protein smoothies in your grocery store's refrigerator to obtain the protein and vitamins you need. Typically, fruit or juice is used to sweeten these beverages. Additionally, you may mix your own protein shakes, giving you complete control over the components. Protein-rich foods that taste good in a smoothie drink include:

• Regular yogurt or Greek yogurt

• Tofu

• Milk

•Tofu milk

• Seeds, nuts, and nut butter

• Powdered dried milk.

Think of blending Greek yogurt, strawberries, bananas, peanut butter, and ice in a blender. Alternately, try tofu with ice, avocado, blueberries, and raspberries.

Making a Protein Shake

1. Start with a base of approximately 1 cup of ice or 1 cup of frozen fruit. Frozen banana is my preferred base, although mixed berries are a close second. It can be put immediately into your powerful mixer.

2. Select your protein source. When producing a protein shake, we often combine several different sources of protein. A serving of protein powder plus a teaspoon each of chia and flax seeds and a tablespoon of nut butter is an example.

3. Sweetener: At this point, select if you want to include a sweetener. You might not need one, depending on the basic fruit you chose or how sweet your protein powder is! If you're going to add one, we advise using a natural sweetener like honey or maple syrup.

4. Liquid: Start with approximately a third to a half cup and add more as needed. Start off cautiously since a

protein shake that is too watery is the worst. Use any beverage you desire, such water, orange juice, almond milk, and so forth.

5. Blend: It's time to combine everything! Your protein smoothie will be smoother the better the blender is. You should add more liquid if something is having trouble "smoothing."

INGREDIENTS

• 1 cup of ice or frozen fruit (banana, berries, etc.)

• 2-4 portions of protein (protein powder, nut butter, seeds, etc.)

• From 1/32 to 1 cup of liquid (almond milk, water, orange juice, etc)

•Sugar is optional

INSTRUCTIONS

1. Fill the bottom of your high-speed blender with ice or fruit first.

2. Add a few of your preferred protein sources after that. Depending on how much protein you want to consume, we advise using 2-4 different sources here.

3. Include 1/3 cup of liquid to begin with and, if preferred, a sweetener.

4. After that, cover your blender and blend on high until the mixture is smooth, about a minute. If your protein shake is having trouble blending, add a little bit additional liquid and blend the mixture again.

5. Serve right away.

Protein Shake with strawberries

What could be better for breakfast than cheesecake? NOTHING! Because it tastes exactly like strawberry cheesecake, you're going to adore this strawberry protein shake. Just a few basic ingredients are needed to make this protein powder smoothie recipe: frozen strawberries, bananas, vanilla protein powder, Greek yogurt, and almond milk. This recipe is incredibly easy to make and tastes just like strawberry cheesecake, whether you call it a strawberry protein shake or a strawberry protein smoothie. You may thank the mixture of Greek yogurt and protein powder for that...creamy and thick.

• Strawberry ice cream

• Bananas frozen

•Grecian yogurt

• Vanilla protein powder (but plain or strawberry also works well!)

• Non-sugared almond milk

Always make sure to blend your protein powder smoothie recipes in a high-speed blender. The secret is to mix everything extremely thoroughly to remove any lumps or bumps.

Smoothie with protein and dates

We used to never add dates to smoothies, but we're here to tell you that doing so is brilliant. It gives a wonderful touch of thickness along with a delightful caramel flavor and a bit of sweetness. Just keep in mind to pit your dates before blending them (been there!). Additionally, if you have a batch of dates that are particularly tough, the simplest method to soften them is to soak them in a cup of water for a few hours, and then you're good to go! Honestly, if you ask me, dates and chocolate go together like a dream.

Ingredients for protein smoothies

This smoothie has protein-rich nut milk (or other milk of your choice) in addition to several other fantastic nutrients, such as:

INGREDIENTS

- 2 medium-sized frozen bananas

- 3 pitted medjool dates

- 1 cup chopped and deboned kale

- 3 tablespoons cocoa powder, dark

- One-half teaspoon of vanilla extract

- 1 cup of your preferred nut milk

INSTRUCTIONS

Blend all the ingredients in a high-speed blender until they are completely smooth.

Use your imagination while choosing the toppings for your smoothie. Here are a few favorites:

- Nutty butters

- The chia seed

- Hemp seedlings

- Sliced Almonds

- Cashews

- Sliced bananas

- Apples in slices

- Blueberries

- Strawberries

- Blackberries

Snack concepts

- Cheese and crackers

- Hummus and pita bread

- Raisin toast, fruit buns, crumpets, fruit buns, scones, muffins, finger buns, or buttered pikelets

- Cream cheese or peanut butter on celery

- cooked eggs;

- Nuts and dried fruits

- Try egg and store-bought mayonnaise, cheese, peanut butter, avocado, tinned salmon, or tuna on toast, sandwiches, or jaffles.

• Milk puddings, including quick puddings, custard, rice pudding, creamed rice, and mousse

• Fruit that has been custard, yoghurt, jelly, ice cream, cream, or condensed milk (fresh, frozen, or canned).

• Fruit stewed with custard or cream.

• Buttery bread and a creamy soup with more cream

• Fish fingers, chicken nuggets, or hot chips

• Veggies frozen in the form of quick noodles

• Corn chips, pretzels, or potato crisps with salsa or guacamole as dips

• Ice cream or yoghurt.

• Sausage rolls, meat pies, samosas, or spring rolls that are frozen

Salads, soups, and vegetables

You may lower your chances of developing cancer, diabetes, hypertension, heart disease, and macular degeneration by consuming five to nine servings of plant-based foods each day. Vitamins, minerals, fiber, phytochemicals, and antioxidants are abundant in fruits and vegetables. Certain fruits and vegetables include antioxidants and phytochemicals that are effective at protecting cells from damage caused by free radicals or other cancer-causing substances.

The following are some suggestions for increasing your intake of fruits and vegetables:

• Having a fruit cocktail for breakfast or sipping fruit or vegetable juice.

• Choosing fruit salad, a piece of fruit, or baby carrots to go with your sandwich rather than potato chips.

• Serving a low-fat garden salad or vegetable soup as an appetizer.

• Stocking up on fruits and veggies in cans, frozen food, and dry form.

• Arranging produce in bowls in the kitchen to make it more aesthetically pleasing.

• Eating dinner with steamed vegetables.

• Bringing pre-washed, chopped fruit and vegetable snacks with you when you go shopping or to work.

Flavored broccoli

The cruciferous vegetable family includes broccoli, cabbage, collard greens, kale, cauliflower, and Brussels sprouts. What a magnificent set of veggies, rich in potent phytochemicals including isothiocyanates, carotenoids, and indoles. Leukemia and melanoma are only two cancers whose growth has been found to be slowed by many of these characteristics, according to research. One substance, indole-3-carbinol, is still being researched because it seems to alter the way estrogen is metabolized, which could inhibit cancer cells from proliferating and expanding as well as halt damaged cells from developing into cancer.

10 minutes for preparation

Cooking Period: 5 minutes

 4 servings.

125 calories, 7.7g total fat (1.1g saturated, 5.4g monounsaturated), 13g carbohydrates, 5g protein, 5g fiber, and 125mg sodium are included in one serving.

Storage: For five to seven days, keep food in the refrigerator in an airtight container.

Ingredients:

1 broccoli bunch

Table salt

Olive oil, extra virgin, two tablespoons

1 tablespoon of garlic, cut coarsely.

12 cup chopped cherry tomatoes or red bell peppers

Red pepper flakes with a pinch

The zest of two lemons

1/4 cup coarsely chopped fresh basil

1 tbsp. of freshly squeezed lemon juice

Cooking Guidelines:

1. Bring a lot of water to a rolling boil. Broccoli stems should be peeled and sliced into bite-sized pieces once the florets have been separated from the stalks. Broccoli stems and florets should be added to the saucepan of water along with a pinch of salt and blanched for 30 seconds. The broccoli will retain its vibrant green color if you drain it and immediately run it under cold water to stop the cooking process.

2. In a sauté pan, heat the olive oil over medium heat. Add the garlic and red pepper flakes, and cook for 30

seconds, or just long enough for the garlic to become aromatic. Add the bell pepper, season with a little salt, and cook for one more minute. After adding the salt, stir in the broccoli florets; the broccoli should still be crisp after 2 minutes. Serve right away after gently incorporating the basil, lemon zest, and juice of the lemon.

Notes:

Basil must be used sparingly! Basil not only has potent antioxidant capabilities, but when mixed with broccoli, peppers, or tomatoes, it significantly amps up the flavor. This recipe is a visual feast thanks to the stunning contrast between the scarlet bell peppers and the brilliant green broccoli. Lemon may dull the color of the broccoli if it rests for more than a few minutes, so be sure to add the juice and zest right before serving.

Almond-studded soup with asparagus and scallions

Serves six

Per serving, there are 146 calories, 24 grams of carbohydrates, 9 grams of protein, 3 grams of fat, 5 grams of fiber, and 304 milligrams of sodium.

NOTE: Without the onion garnish, this recipe is suitable for persons following the Low Microbial Diet (LMD). If dairy consumption is restricted, lactose-free milk may be used instead.

Ingredients:

1/4 cup of chopped almonds for decoration

1 tablespoon olive oil

To taste, 1/2 tsp. dried thyme

2 medium leeks, finely cut, with the white part only

1 can (15 oz.) of washed and drained cannellini white beans

2 cans of fat-free, low-sodium chicken broth, each weighing 14 ounces

To taste, add salt and white pepper.

1 tablespoon Low-sodium soy sauce

6 thinly sliced scallions, plus 2 for garnish

2 pounds of asparagus (stem ends trimmed)

A single cup of evaporated skim milk (optional)

*After puréeing and pouring back into the saucepan, mix in 1 cup evaporated skim milk for a creamier soup. Ladle into serving dishes after heating.

Cooking Guidelines:

1. Place almonds in a saucepan over medium heat if using as a garnish. 5 to 6 minutes of toasting, stirring regularly to prevent scorching, until nuts are golden. Put nuts on paper towels and set them aside.

2. Heat the oil in the same pan at a medium heat. Include 4 chopped scallions and leeks. Cook for 5–6 minutes, stirring periodically, or until vegetables are soft. Bring to a boil the broth, thyme, salt, and pepper. Include beans and asparagus. Bring to a boil once more, then immediately lower heat and simmer, partially covered, for 12 to 15 minutes, or until veggies are tender. Remove from heat and allow it cool a little.

3. Use a blender to fully blend the soup. Refill the saucepan and heat it up to medium. Warm through. Put Into serving bowls and ladle. Add the remaining scallions and toast some almonds as garnish.

Corn and Black Bean Salad

Enjoy with tortillas made with maize or whole wheat and add shrimp!

This salad works well as a side dish for Mexican main dishes or as a dipping sauce for tortilla chips before the dinner. Feel free to experiment while using the measurements as a guide. When you have leftover corn on the cob, keep this salad in mind.

15 minutes or less in total

Servings: 8

Serving size: 20 grams of total carbohydrates, 7 grams of dietary fiber, 0 mg of cholesterol, 6 grams of protein, 2.5 grams of total fat, and 125 calories.

Ingredients:

1 diced tomatoes

Chopped red onion, half a small one

Freshly ground black pepper and salt

14 cup freshly chopped cilantro

2 (15-ounce) cans of rinsed and drained black beans

1 cup drained no-salt-added fresh, frozen, or canned corn

2 teaspoons of fresh lime juice

1 tbsp. Olive oil

1 teaspoon of cumin, ground

1 seeded and coarsely chopped jalapeno

1 chopped and seeded red, yellow, or green bell pepper

Cooking Guidelines:

Black beans, corn, tomato, bell pepper, onion, and jalapeo should all be combined in a bowl.

2. Drizzle the bean mixture with the mixture of lime juice, oil, and cumin in a bowl. Add cilantro and season with salt and pepper.

Apple and Carrot Soup

Serves four

132 calories, 23 grams of carbohydrates, 4 grams of protein, 4 grams of fat (0 grams of saturated fat), 5 grams of fiber, and 496 milligrams of sodium are contained in one serving.

NOTE: If you are limited from dairy, substitute lactose-free milk if you'd like. This dish is acceptable for individuals on the LMD (Low Microbial Diet) without the mint garnish.

Ingredients:

1 chopped medium onion

One small leek, chopped

1 pound of peeled, thinly sliced carrots

3 cups of low-fat, sodium-reduced chicken broth

1 chopped, peeled, and cored Granny Smith apple

1 teaspoon canola oil

To taste, add salt and freshly ground black pepper.

Mint, minced, 3 tablespoons, for garnish (optional)

If desired, add more broth or fat-free milk (optional)

Cooking Guidelines:

1. In a medium Dutch oven or big saucepan, heat the oil until it is hot. Cook the onion and leek for about 4 minutes, or until the onion is transparent.

2. Combine apple and carrots. Cook veggies gently for 8 to 10 minutes, with a tight lid on the pot and the heat reduced. Add broth. Carrots should be very soft after around 30 minutes of cooking under cover.

3. Allow the soup to sit, uncovered, for around 20 minutes to gently cool. If required, puree the soup in two batches in a blender or food processor. (A soup using a blender is smoother.) Add more milk or broth, as desired, if the soup is too thick. Use salt and pepper to taste to season. Serve with mint as a garnish.

Sweet Potato Lentil Soup

Almost any cuisine pairs well with sweet potatoes. Lentils and sweet potatoes combine to form a delectable soup in this dish.

25 minutes for preparation

50 minutes to cook (majority of cooking time requires minimal monitoring)

Serves four

380 calories, 45 grams of carbs, 18.5 grams of protein, 14 grams of fat, and 15 grams of fiber are included in one serving.

NOTE: If black pepper is left out at the end, it's acceptable for people following the Low Microbial Diet.

Ingredients:

2 tbsp. olive oil

1 tbsp. sesame oil

2 big, chopped red onions

1 1/2 tsp. dried thyme

4 minced garlic cloves (to save time, you can use minced garlic in a jar)

Vegetable stock in 10 cups (to save time, use vegetarian bouillon cubes, or boxed stock; omit salt if you use boullion)

Green, brown, or red lentils, 1 1/4 cups

2 cup celery stalks

12 cup split, freshly minced parsley

To taste, freshly ground pepper

1 pound of two medium sweet potatoes, diced and peeled

12 teaspoon of salt (omit salt if you use bouillon instead of fresh vegetable stock)

Cooking Guidelines:

1. Heat the olive and sesame oils in a large pot over medium-high heat. The onion, lightly stir while sautéing until onions are tender (5-7 minutes).

2. Include thyme and garlic. Cook for a further 2 to 3 minutes. Don't cook garlic too long. Reduce heat if browning occurs with the garlic.

3. Turn up the heat all the way. Add 14 cup of the parsley, the stock, the lentils, and the celery.

4. Heat mixture to a simmer after bringing it to a boil.

5. Cook for 30 minutes uncovered.

6. Add the sweet potatoes and simmer for a further 20 minutes, or until they are fork-tender.

7. Take 2 cups of the soup out and mix it. Blend thoroughly till thick and smooth. Be extremely cautious during blending, and remove the lid of the blender slowly every few seconds to let steam and heat escape. The blender's lid may come off if there is a buildup of

steam and heat (skip the blender step if thinner soup is desired).

8. Add the remaining 1/4 cup of parsley to the pot along with the blended soup. Stir and mix for the final minute of cooking.

9. Taste-test and add freshly ground pepper.

10. Dish out and savor!

Salad of Pomegranates

Serves six

92 calories, 5g fat (less than 1g saturated), 14g carbohydrates, 1g protein, 2g fiber, and 9mg sodium per serving.

NOTE: LMD patients should NOT attempt this recipe (Low Microbial Diet).

Ingredients:

2 tablespoons lime juice, fresh

2 tbsp. olive oil

Pomegranate seeds in a half-cup (from 1 med pomegranate)

Arugula in 2 medium bunches, thoroughly cleaned and stems cut off.

2 ripe but firm pears, sliced in half, cored, and into 6 wedges each.

1/2 Dijon mustard

Freshly ground black pepper and salt

12 cup feta cheese crumbles (optional)

Toasted and roughly chopped 1/3 cup pecans (optional)

18 Bibb, Boston, or green-leafed lettuce leaves that have been rinsed and dried (optional)

Cooking Guidelines:

1. To make dressing, combine lime juice, oil, and mustard in a small bowl.

2. Add arugula and pears to a salad bowl. Add just enough dressing to coat and toss. Use salt and pepper to taste to season. Serve the dish garnished with feta, pecans (if used), and pomegranate seeds. Alternately, arrange lettuce leaves on the bottom of each salad plate and pile the salad on top.

Vegetable soup

Servings of vegetable soup: (8) Each Serving: 3g fat, 32g carbohydrates, 15g protein, 5mg chol, and high fiber make up 215 calories.

NOTE: This meal is suitable for individuals on the LMD (Low Microbial Diet), however the vegetables must be well cooked and no pepper should be added thereafter. To your taste, you can add any number of vegetable combinations.

Ingredients:

1 big, chopped onion

1 tablespoon of margarine or butter

1 sweet potato, chopped after peeling

2 white potatoes, diced after being peeled

2 big carrots, chopped after being peeled

2 big, sliced zucchini

1 cup of Green beans

4-6 cups of beef or chicken broth

2 cups chopped broccoli florets

1 cup of Green peas

1/4 tsp. paprika

Pepper and salt as desired

Cooking Guidelines:

1. Melt butter in a frying pan and sauté onions until they are transparent.

2. Place onions, sweet potatoes, white potatoes, carrots, zucchini, and beans in a large soup pot.

3. Include broth.

3. Heat to a boil.

5. Turn down the heat, cover, and simmer for about 30 minutes.

6. Paprika, broccoli, and peas should be added 10 minutes before serving.

7. Add salt to taste. If preferred, the soup may be blended in a blender or food processor.

Chicken, papaya, and pecan salad

This spring, add a fresh spin to your salad. Both dietary fiber and vitamin C are packed into this meal. Enjoy! (Or use mango instead!)

Serves four

220 calories, 11g fat (1g saturated fat), 17g carbohydrates, 16g protein, 4g fiber, and 62mg sodium are contained in one serving.

NOTE: LMD users are not permitted (Low Microbial Diet).

Ingredients:

1 medium papaya or mango, cut in half, seeded, peeled, and cubed (approximately 1 /12 cups).

Half-pound of skinless, boneless chicken breasts

4 cups romaine lettuce, torn

½ Dijon mustard

1 /12 Tbsp. olive oil

14 cup toasted pecan halves

To taste, add salt and freshly ground black pepper.

Red pepper slices in one cup (about 1 large pepper)

2 thinly sliced onions (about 1/4 cup)

2 tbsp. of Red wine vinegar

A tablespoon of lime juice

1 teaspoon honey

1 water cup

1 minced garlic clove (approximately 12 tsp.)

Cooking Guidelines:

1. Bring 1 cup of water to a boil in a 10 inch nonstick skillet. Cook the chicken breasts after adding them. Cook for about 15 minutes, covered, over low heat, or until chicken is thoroughly cooked.

2. Transfer the chicken to a covered container using a slotted spoon. In the refrigerator, cool.

3. Combine lettuce, papaya, red pepper, and scallions in a big salad dish. Mix the vinegar, lime juice, honey, garlic, and mustard in a measuring cup. Add oil gradually in a thin stream. Blender is well-whisked.

4. Taste-test and add salt and pepper. Combine chicken with dressing after cutting it into bite-sized pieces. Mix

the lettuce with the chicken and dressing. Put pecans on top.

Salad of feta cheese, red bell pepper, and spinach with yogurt dressing

Serves six

41 calories, 1 g fat, 6 g carbohydrates, 2 g protein, 91 mcg sodium, and 1 g fiber are included in one serving.

NOTE: People on the LMD should avoid making this recipe (Low Microbial Diet).

Ingredients:

12 cup plain nonfat yogurt

1 teaspoon of honey

2 tablespoons of chopped dill

1 big chopped red bell pepper (about 1 cup)

1 bag (5 oz) of finely chopped baby spinach (about 4 cups)

Black pepper freshly ground

1 celery stalk, cut into dice (about 1 cup)

14 cup of green onions, finely sliced (scallions)

1 oz. of crumbled, washed, and drained feta cheese (equivalent to 1/4 cup)

Cooking Guidelines:

1. Stir the yogurt, honey, dill, and black pepper together in a large basin.

2. Stir in the spinach, red pepper, celery, and green onions.

3. Feta cheese is added before serving.

Salad of salmon with herbs and pimento

Serves six

140 calories, 9g fat, 2g saturated fat, 14g protein, 341mg sodium, and 2g carbohydrates are contained in one serving.

NOTE: People on the LMD should avoid making this recipe (Low Microbial Diet).

Ingredients:

1 cup of celery, diced

¼ cup of minced White onion

1 jar (2 oz) of drained, chopped pimentos

Two to three teaspoons of low-fat mayonnaise

1 can (14 oz) of well-drained, skin- and bone-free red salmon;

OR 14 oz. fresh cooked salmon

1 tablespoon of lemon juice, fresh

One tablespoon of fresh dill

1/4 paprika teaspoon (optional)

Pepper, freshly ground, to taste

10 capers, 1 tablespoon (optional)

Either 2 teaspoons of dried chives or 2 tablespoons of fresh chives

Cooking Guidelines:

1. Combine salmon with celery, onion, and pimentos in a medium bowl.

2. Combine mayonnaise, lemon juice, chives, dill, optional paprika, and black pepper in a small bowl. Add to salmon mixture.

3. Add capers to the top and serve right away with whole wheat pita wedges, if preferred.

Delicious Brown Rice and Vegetable Soup

Serves five

73 calories, 11 grams of carbohydrates, 5 grams of protein, 1 gram of fat (less than 1 gram of saturated fat), 2 grams of fiber, and 481 milligrams of sodium are contained in one serving.

NOTE: If all of the ingredients and cheese are heated into the soup, this recipe is suitable for people on the LMD (Low Microbial Diet).

- Use lactose-free cheese if you must avoid dairy products.

Ingredients:

12 cup of brown rice in a bag

Chopped broccoli florets, 1 cup

Chopped cauliflower florets, 1 cup

1 finely sliced carrot

2 cans of fat-free, low-sodium chicken broth (15 oz each).

1 teaspoon dried basil

Dried oregano, 1 teaspoon

1 tsp. dried ground cumin

To taste, add salt and freshly ground pepper.

Grated cheese, half a cup (romano or parmesan)

Cooking Guidelines:

1. Bring broth to a boil in a big pot. Add brown rice and stir. For five minutes, cook with a cover over low heat.

2. Include oregano and veggies. For about 5 minutes, simmer, or until the vegetables are soft.

3. Include the cumin, basil, salt, and pepper. Pour soup into dishes and top with cheese shavings.

Irish cream soup

This St. Patrick's Day, think green, think cabbage, and think wholesome. This revised version of a hearty, nutritious cabbage soup will help you spread a little luck of the Irish. On St. Patrick's Day, cabbage has always been a staple on an Irish dinner, as it should be. The polyphenols, fiber, and vitamins C and A found in cabbage give it the ability to help fight cancer. Any dinner would be a terrific place to start with this soup.

Serves five (1 cup each)

125 calories, 2g of saturated fat, 17g of total carbohydrates, 7g of protein, 2g of dietary fiber, and 295mg of sodium are contained in one serving.

NOTE: As long as NO GARNISH is added, this recipe is OK for individuals following the LMD (Low Microbial Diet). For individuals who are permitted dairy, you may top the dish with processed Parmesan cheese.

Ingredients:

1-12-pound cabbage, quartered and cored

1 tbsp. Canola oil

12 cup potato, diced and peeled

Tightly packed half a cup of light brown sugar

1/2 cup of flour

1 teaspoon freshly chopped chive

To taste, add salt and pepper.

2 cups of low-fat, sodium-reduced chicken broth.

Hot water

1 chopped medium onion

2 tbsp. Canola oil

14–12 teaspoons of powdered nutmeg

2 cups of milk with 2 percent reduced fat

2 tbsp. grated Parmesan cheese

1 tbsp. Chopped fresh flat-leaf parsley

Cooking Guidelines:

1. Fill a big bowl with cabbage. Cover the cabbage with a layer of boiling water. Give the cabbage five minutes to soak in the water. Good drainage then chop the cabbage into thin pieces after patting it dry using paper towels.

2. Fill a sizable, heavy saucepan with canola oil. The onions should be sautéed until soft but not browned (about 10 minutes). Cook the potato cubes and cabbage for 5 minutes while stirring. Stir for two minutes after adding the flour and nutmeg.

3. Gradually incorporate the broth and milk. Stirring often, bring it to a boil. For about 20 minutes, reduce

the heat and cook the vegetables until they are soft. Give it some time to cool.

4. Use a blender or food processor to puree the soup in batches, if required, until it is smooth. Add salt and pepper, and then put the soup back in the pot. Simmer it for a while, and then ladle it into bowls and top with Parmesan, chives, and parsley.

Main dishes and side dishes

Butternut Squash, Turkey, and Barley Casserole

Eating in a healthy manner is simple with this one-pot dinner. A wonderful treat for Thanksgiving!

Serves six

275 calories, 5g fat (2g saturated), 42g carbohydrate, 18g protein, 10g fiber, and 368mg sodium are contained in one serving.

NOTE: People on the LMD can make this recipe (Low Microbial Diet).

Ingredients:

Utilize baking pans without sticking or cooking spray.

2 cups of low-sodium, fat-free chicken broth

2 little butternut squash

Quick-cooking barley, 1/4 cup

12 pound cooked, chopped, or cut up turkey breast

1 chopped and seeded green bell pepper

1 teaspoon olive oil

12 cup feta cheese crumbles

12 cup of minced onion

Dry sage, 1 teaspoon

Pepper, freshly ground, to taste

Cooking Guidelines:

1. Set oven to 350 degrees. Use a non-stick dish or spray cooking spray to coat a 4-quart baking dish.

2. Boil squash halves for five minutes or until almost cooked in a big pot of quickly boiling water. Drain. Scoop the flesh from each half and dice it after it is cool enough to handle. Place aside.

3. Heat oil in a big pot over medium heat. Add the cubed squash, green pepper, and onion. 3 minutes of sauté. Stir in the pepper and sage after adding them. Bring to a boil after adding broth. Back to boiling after adding barley.

4. Reduce heat to low, cover the pot, and simmer the barley for 10 minutes, or until the liquid has been absorbed. Mix in the turkey cubes. Add feta cheese on top after transferring the mixture to the prepared baking dish. Bake uncovered for 30 minutes or until golden cheese.

Baked Bean and Vegetable Enchilada

Servings: 8

320 calories, 2g of saturated fat, 53g of carbs, 15g of protein, 11g of dietary fiber, and 677mg of sodium are included in one serving.

NOTE: Safe for anyone following a low-microbiome diet.

Ingredients:

1 can (14 oz.) rinsed and drain black beans

1 chopped medium bell pepper

1 big, chopped onion

2 minced garlic cloves

Canola oil, 1 tablespoon

1 package (16 ounces) of thawed frozen corn

28 ounces of crushed or pureed tomatoes in one can

1 can (14 oz.) washed and drain pinto beans

Chili powder, 1 tablespoon

12 tsp. cumin powder

Spicy sauce, to taste, in a dash

To taste, add salt and freshly ground pepper.

12 corn tortillas

1 cup shredded Jack cheese with less fat

Cooking Guidelines:

1. Set oven to 350 degrees. For five minutes, sauté bell pepper, onion, and garlic in oil in a large skillet over medium heat. Beans, corn, tomatoes, and seasonings (salt, pepper, as preferred) can all be added. Simmer for 15 minutes on low heat.

2. Put the casserole together in a 9 x 13-inch baking pan. Add one-third of the bean mixture to the bottom. Beans are covered with six tortilla layers. Continue, finishing with bean mixture on top. 30 to 40 minutes later, cover with cheese and bake until cheese is melted and bubbling.

Beans surprise

One of the healthiest foods available is beans, which are also referred to as legumes. Research repeatedly demonstrates that those who regularly include more beans in their diet have a lower chance of developing heart disease and cancer. In fact, a recent study found that women who consume beans or lentils two or more times per week have a significant 24 percent lower risk of developing breast cancer than those who consume them less frequently. Beans should undoubtedly play a significant role in any diet designed to combat cancer. This meal might not be suitable for you if you are undergoing cancer treatment and are having trouble eating enough to maintain your weight because beans can be highly filling and result in bloating and gas. For a delicious supper, serve with a side of steamed vegetables, a fruit salad, or a fresh green salad.

Serves four

225 calories, 38 grams of carbohydrates, 11 grams of protein, 6 grams of fat, and 9 grams of fiber are included in each serving.

NOTE: Without the yogurt and with properly cooked vegetables, this recipe is suitable for individuals following the Low Microbial Diet.

Ingredients:

15-ounce can of black beans

1 teaspoon olive oil

2 teaspoons yellow mustard

4 large tortillas, whole wheat or sprouted wheat

1 teaspoon cumin (dried spice)

2 teaspoons of low-sodium soy sauce

4 oz. of shredded soy or rice cheese in the form of mozzarella

Cooking Guidelines:

1. Thoroughly rinse and drain the black beans. You may lessen the amount of gas you might get from eating beans by rinsing the liquid off of canned beans.

2. In a pan over medium heat, combine black beans, cumin, olive oil, low sodium soy sauce, and yellow mustard.

3. While the ingredients are heating, stir the beans.

4. Slightly mash the beans to make the mixture a little bit "stickier."

5. Split the bean mixture into four equal halves, and then arrange one on each side of the large tortilla shell.

6. Top the beans on each tortilla with 1 oz of shredded soy or rice cheese.

7. Add a small amount of olive oil—about 1 teaspoon— and coat a flat skillet with it. Stir fry pan over medium heat.

8. To make a half circle, fold the tortilla in half and press to make the two halves stick together.

9. Place the tortillas in the skillet and warm them on both sides (flip once). Heat the tortilla just long enough for the cheese to melt.

10. Add plain low-fat yogurt as a garnish. Enjoy & Serve!

Spaghetti alla carbonara

Each serving of traditional carbonara typically has 574 calories and 27 grams of fat. With the updated recipe, only 307 calories and 7 grams of fat are produced.

Time Spent Preparing and Cooking: 40 minutes

6 servings

307 calories, 7g fat, 2g saturated fat, 45g carbohydrates, 19g protein, 8g fiber, 121mg cholesterol, and 528mg sodium are contained in one serving.

NOTE: As long as all of the vegetables AND the cheese are thoroughly cooked, this meal is suitable for persons following the Low Microbial Diet. For individuals who cannot have dairy, omit the cheese.

Ingredients:

Extra-virgin olive oil, 1 teaspoon

2 minced garlic cloves

A quarter cup of low-sodium chicken broth

Three big eggs

8 ounces of stemmed, quartered, and diced broccolini or broccoli rabe, depending on the amount being used.

3 ounces (12 cup) of diced, thinly sliced prosciutto or Canadian bacon.

Freshly ground pepper, 1/4 teaspoon

Salt as desired

12 ounces of whole-wheat pasta or spaghetti

Pinch of red pepper flakes (optional)

A third cup of freshly grated Romano or Parmesan cheese (for a lactose free diet, choose lactose free cheese)

Cooking Guidelines:

1. Start a big pot of water to boil for pasta. Additionally, heat the bottom of a double boiler with about 1 inch of water to a moderate simmer (don't have a double boiler? Instead, place a sizzling water pan over a big stainless steel bowl.

2. In a medium nonstick skillet, heat the oil over medium heat. Add the prosciutto (or Canadian bacon) and cook,

turning often, for 2 minutes or until heated through. Add the crushed red pepper and garlic, and stir-fry for 30 seconds. Get rid of the heat.

3. In the top of the double boiler, whisk together the eggs, broth, and pepper. Set in the bottom of a double boiler over simmering water, and cook for 5-7 minutes, whisking continuously in a slow, steady figure-eight motion, until the sauce steams and thickens enough to coat a metal spoon. There might be a few little curdles in the sauce. To prevent the sauce from continuing to curdle, turn off the heat under the top pan and quickly whisk the mixture.

4. In the meantime, cook the pasta in the boiling water for 5 minutes, tossing often. Add broccolini (or broccoli rabe) and continue cooking for an additional 4-6 minutes or until the pasta is cooked but firm. Place the drained food in a big bowl. Add the cheese, prosciutto (or bacon) mixture, and egg sauce and combine thoroughly. Adding salt is optional.

Grilled Vegetable Polenta with Tomato Sauce and Pan-Roasted Red Pepper

244 calories, 11g fat, 2g saturated fat, 450mg salt, and 2mg cholesterol per serving.

NOTE: If you're following the Low Microbial Diet, omit the parsley from this recipe.

Polenta ingredients:

½ tbsp. basil leaves

A little pepper

14 cup red onion, diced

1 zucchini, chopped

34 tsp. fresh garlic, chopped

1 chopped red pepper, chopped

Tbsp. of olive oil

12 oz. Grated parmesan

Dash of salt

4.4 ounces of cornmeal

8 oz. of water

8 ounces of veggie broth

Polenta Cooking Instructions:

1. Set the oven's temperature to 350.

2. Combine the salt, pepper, garlic, and dried basil. Vegetables should be cut in half and spiced.

3. Use the olive oil to grease a cookie sheet. Place the vegetables on the grill and cook for 10–12 minutes, or until they are tender. If you don't have a grill, you may simply bake them in the oven at the same time.

4. Add salt and polenta after bringing broth and water to a boil. until the polenta is smooth, constantly stir

5. Combine cooked vegetables and cheese. Place in a pan and bake for 10 minutes at 350 degrees F.

6. Use a biscuit cutter to cut the dough into squares or circles. Serve with sauce right away (recipe below).

Red pepper/tomato sauce ingredients:

3 tablespoons of olive oil

3 Roma Tomatoes

1 cup of soup

Red Peppers, two (seeded)

4 cloves of chopped garlic

Salt, as desired

Pepper, as desired

Parley (topper)

Cooking Directions for Sauce

1. Warm pan to a high temperature.

2. Add oil and tomatoes; as soon as the tomatoes begin to caramelize and turn black; scrape the bottom of the pan.

3. Add the garlic and red bell peppers, and simmer for an additional five minutes.

4. Remove the veggies from the pan and add broth to deglaze it.

5. Use a spatula to remove the vegetables that have caramelized on the pan's bottom.

6. In a food processor or blender, combine this mixture with the cooked veggies and purée until completely smooth.

7. Add pepper and salt to taste.

8. Add parsley to the top of the polenta circles or squares.

Southwestern-style soft tacos with vegetables

These vegetarian soft tacos are topped with salsa and filled with sauteed vegetables. Serve it as a meal with Spanish rice, melon cubes, and a green salad toss with red wine vinegar dressing.

Serves four

Two tacos provide 295 calories, 6g of fat (1g saturated), 55g of carbohydrates, 10g of protein, 10g of fiber, 0 mg of cholesterol, and 221mg of sodium per serving.

NOTE: If the veggies are properly cooked and the salsa is from a jar, this recipe is suitable for anyone following the Low Microbial Diet. AVOID FRESH CILANTRO!

Ingredients:

1 tablespoon olive oil

1 chopped medium red onion

1 cup of yellow summer squash, chopped.

1 cup of green zucchini dice

Chop and seed 4 medium tomatoes.

1 cup washed and drained canned pinto or black beans

Minced three big garlic cloves

A single seeded and sliced jalapeño chili

Chopped fresh cilantro, half a cup

8 Corn tortillas

1 cup of frozen corn or 1 cup of fresh corn kernels

12 cup salsa with a smoky flavor (or regular flavored)

Cooking Guidelines:

1. Heat the olive oil in a big pot over medium heat. Cook the onion after adding it till tender. Cook the zucchini and summer squash after adding them for about 5 more minutes, or until they are tender. Add the beans, corn kernels, garlic, tomatoes, and jalapenos after stirring. Cook for about 5 minutes, or until the vegetables are crisp-tender. After adding the cilantro, turn off the heat.

2. Set a dry, sizable frying pan with a medium heat and a nonstick surface. One tortilla should be added to the hot

pan and heated for 20 seconds on each side until tender. Repeat with the remaining tortillas.

3. Distribute the tortillas among individual dishes before serving. On each tortilla, evenly distribute the veggie mixture. Add 2 tablespoons of the salsa on the top of each. Serve right away.

Italian Chicken Stir Fry in 10 Minutes

Serves four

316 calories, 7g of fat (1g saturated), 27g of carbohydrates, 6g of fiber, 27g of protein, and 244mg of sodium are contained in each serving.

Ingredients:

1 tbsp. extra virgin olive oil

12 cup freshly cut pre-sliced mushrooms

1 teaspoon minced garlic, fine

1-teaspoon dried basil

1 tbsp. Dried oregano

1 frozen 16-ounce bag of mixed vegetables (or 3-4 cups fresh chopped vegetables)

2 cups of brown rice, cooked

Grated Parmesan cheese, two tablespoons

To taste, add salt and freshly ground black pepper.

12 cup chicken broth with less salt and fat

34 lb., 34 inch-long, boneless, skinless chicken breast

Cooking Guidelines:

First, make brown rice. During the rice's cooking, heat a sizable pan on high. Oil is added, stirred to coat the pan, and heated until extremely hot.

2. Stir-fry the chicken once it has lost its pink hue. Remove the chicken from the pan using a slotted spoon and set it aside.

3. Fill the pan with vegetables and garlic. Stir-fry for about 2 minutes, or until garlic is aromatic.

4. Include mushrooms. Add 2 more minutes of stirring and return chicken back into the pan.

5. Add chicken broth, basil, and oregano.

6. Stir-fry for a further 4 minutes or until chicken is completely cooked.

7. Stir in the cheese. Use salt and pepper to taste. Serve immediately with pan juices over the brown rice.

Bok Choy with Shallots and Sautéed Mushrooms

Serve this meal with grilled fish and brown rice (optional).

Serves four

65 calories, 1g of saturated fat, 8g of carbohydrates, 4g of protein, 2g of fiber, and 213mg of sodium are included in one serving.

NOTE: If you exclude the lemon zest and pepper from this dish, it is OK for individuals following the Low Microbial Diet.

Ingredients:

1 package of sliced mushrooms (8 oz).

2 tablespoons canola or olive oil

2 minced shallots

Bok choy, 1 1/2 pounds, washed, and cut into 1-inch pieces.

1 minced garlic clove

2 teaspoons of light soy sauce

1-teaspoon lemon zest

To taste, add salt and freshly ground pepper.

Cooking Guidelines:

1. Heat oil in a big skillet or wok over a high heat. Stir-fry the mushrooms, shallots, and garlic for about five minutes, or until the mushrooms turn black.

2. Stir-fry the bok choy for 8 to 10 minutes, or until it is soft. Add salt, pepper, soy sauce, and lemon zest.

3. Serve.

Garlic-seasoned spinach

An excellent supply of iron, magnesium, potassium, folate, vitamin A, and vitamin C.

40 minutes total for preparation and cooking

4 servings of 1/2 cup each.

Per serving, there are 72 calories, 4g of fat, 1g of saturated fat, 4g of protein, 258mg of sodium, 6g of carbohydrates, and 3g of fiber.

NOTE: As long as the veggies are well cooked, this meal is suitable for individuals following the LMD (Low Microbial Diet).

Ingredients:

2 minced garlic cloves

1 teaspoon oil from toasted sesame

1 bag of spinach weighing 10 ounces, with stems cut off

1 chopped and trimmed scallion

4 grains of salt (optional)

1 teaspoon of roasted sesame seeds*, plus extras for decoration.

Sesame seeds should be lightly toasted for 3-5 minutes in a small, dry skillet over medium-high heat while stirring regularly.

Cooking Instructions:

1. Start by heating up a sizable kettle of water. Just until the spinach turns brilliant green, around 30 seconds, add

the spinach and stir. Drain and quickly rinse under cold water. Squeeze extra water out.

2. In a big skillet, heat the oil over medium-high heat. Stirring constantly, add the garlic and simmer for 30 to 60 seconds or until fragrant. Add the spinach, scallion, sesame seeds, and salt after removing from the heat (if desired). To blend, stir. To allow the flavors to permeate the spinach, allow to stand for around 10 minutes. Serve warm or cold with more toasted sesame seeds on top.

Winter Caponata

Serves: 10 (½ cup per serving)

80 calories, 4.5g fat (less than 1g saturated), 10g carbohydrates, 2g protein, 2g fiber, and 90mg sodium are included in one serving.

Ingredients:

Small broccoli florets, 4 cups

Divided 2 tablespoons of extra virgin olive oil

1 chopped medium onion

1 celery stalk, finely sliced

1 minced garlic clove

Remove the stems and center vein from 1 bunch of Swiss chard and cut the leaves into 34-inch strips.

1/4 Low-sodium tomato sauce

¼ cup of Raisins

2 tbsp. Red wine vinegar

1 teaspoon sugar

3 tablespoons pine nuts

1 tablespoon of washed and drained capers

Asian eggplant weighing 12 kg, chopped into 1-inch pieces

Cooking Guidelines:

1. Steam the broccoli and chard until they are soft and lightly browned over water. One tablespoon of oil has been heated to medium-high heat in a medium skillet. Add the onion and cook for approximately 5 minutes, or until it begins to brown. After adding the last of the oil, stack the eggplant slices in the pan. 3 minutes to cook. Become the slices with tongs and heat for another 3 minutes, or until the eggplant is just starting to turn light

brown. Add the tomato sauce, raisins, celery, and garlic. Steamed veggies should then be added and combined. Cook covered over low heat for 10 minutes, tossing periodically, until the broccoli is very tender. In the meantime, mix the vinegar and sugar in a small basin. To the skillet, add them. Cook for 2 minutes, stirring three or four times, after adding the pine nuts and capers. Use salt and pepper to taste to season.

2. Spoon the caponata into a bowl and leave it there to cool to room temperature. Serve right away, or cover and chill until you're ready to. When kept in a refrigerator with a tight lid, caponata lasts for five days.

Rice with Tofu

Serves four

376 calories, 11g fat (2g saturated), 50g carbohydrates, 3.2g fiber, 16g protein, 106mg cholesterol, and 629mg sodium are contained in one serving.

NOTE: As long as all veggies are well cooked, this meal is suitable for individuals following the LMD (Low Microbial Diet).

Ingredients:

Rice, two cups (preferably brown)

2 tablespoons vegetable oil, split

12 teaspoon dark sesame oil

2 big, lightly beaten eggs

1 cup of sliced green onions

1 14-ounce package of firm tofu with little fat, drained, and cubed

2 teaspoons of prepared garlic mince

1 teaspoon canned fresh ginger minced

2 tablespoons sake, an optional rice wine

Low-sodium soy sauce, 3 tablespoons

1-tablespoon hoisin sauce

1 cup of fresh or frozen carrots and peas

Cooking Guidelines:

1. Prepare rice. Leave out the salt and the fat.

2. Heat 1 tablespoon of vegetable oil in a big nonstick skillet over medium-high heat while the rice is cooking. Add the tofu and cook, stirring periodically, for 4

minutes or until lightly browned. Take out of pan. Add eggs to the pan and cook for one minute, breaking them up as they cook. Take out of pan. Pan with 1 Tbsp of vegetable oil. Add a cup of onions, carrots, peas, and ginger; sauté for two minutes.

3. Combine sake, soy sauce, hoisin sauce, and sesame oil while the vegetable mixture cooks. Add the cooked rice to the pan and stir continuously for 2 minutes. Add the tofu, egg, and soy sauce combination and stir continuously for 30 seconds.

Grilled Portobello Mushrooms

Serves four

Per Serving: Each serving has 39 calories, 2g fat (0 g saturated), 4g carbs, 2g fiber, 2g protein, 0mg chol, 89mg sodium

Ingredients:

Olive oil, 1 1/2 Tbsp

1 tsp chopped fresh basil

Black pepper freshly ground

1 1/2 cloves of minced garlic

Salt, as desired

Four Portobello mushrooms

Cooking Guidelines:

1. Light the grill.

2. Combine the olive oil, garlic, salt, and pepper.

3. Cut the mushroom stems off, then brush the olive oil mixture on both sides of the caps. Place aside.

4. Grill the mushrooms for 3 to 4 minutes on each side, or until they are tender throughout.

5. Transfer to a cutting board and slice into 1 inch strips.

Pilaf of butternut squash

Serves six

Per Serving: 201 calories, 35g carbohydrates, 5g protein, 5g fat, 1g saturated fat, 4g fiber, and 199mg sodium.

NOTE: If the parsley, cranberries, salt, and pepper are cooked in or left out, this recipe is suitable for people on the LMD (Low Microbial Diet).

Ingredients:

1 teaspoon olive oil

12 cup of minced onion

2 minced garlic cloves

1/4 cup of almonds, sliced

1 teaspoon cumin, ground (optional)

2 cups of fat-free or reduced-sodium vegetable or chicken broth

1 serving brown rice

2 Tbsp. freshly chopped parsley

12 ounces of dried cranberries

To taste, add salt and pepper.

Dried oregano, 1 teaspoon

3 cups of butternut squash, chopped and peeled

Cooking Guidelines:

1. Heat the oil in a medium saucepan over a medium-high heat. Sauté the onion and garlic for 2 minutes, or until tender.

2. Stir in the almonds and heat for 1–2 minutes, or until golden. Add rice, cumin and oregano and stir to cool. Add broth and bring to boil.

3. Lower the heat to low, cover the pan and boil the rice for 30 minutes or until it is

4. Remove from the heat and toss in the cranberries and parsley. To taste, add salt and pepper to the dish.

Anti-cancer ketogenic diet

The ketogenic diet, which is high in fat and protein and low in carbohydrates, appears to make most malignancies more responsive to standard therapy by taking advantage of the altered metabolism of cancer cells. This makes the diet a prospective choice for adjuvant cancer therapy. The ketogenic diet might be thought of as a promising adjuvant as a patient-specific multifactorial therapy since it likely generates an unfavorable metabolic environment for cancer cells. Based on its potential to enhance the antitumor effects of conventional chemo- and radiotherapy, its general good safety and tolerability, and its potential to improve quality of life, the majority of preclinical and a few clinical studies support the use of the ketogenic diet in combination with standard therapies. However, further molecular research as well as rigorously controlled clinical trials are required to better understand the mechanics of the ketogenic diet as a treatment and assess its use in clinical practice.

The keto diet is "neutral" on protein and high in fat (55 to 60 percent), low in carbohydrates (5 to 10 percent). It does frequently contain a little bit more protein than the normal Western diet, at 30% to 35% of all calories. The ketogenic diet aims to burn fat as the body's main fuel source rather than sugar. The body changes to burning fat, which results in the production of ketone bodies, when carbohydrate consumption is drastically reduced. We refer to this as keto-adaptation.

Effects of Cancer Cell

Based on what fuels cancer cells, one theory on how keto might function postulates that it might restrict cancer cells' growth by effectively "starving" them. This area of science is not at all novel: The discovery of the Warburg effect by scientist Otto Warburg earned him the 1931 Nobel Prize in Physiology and Medicine. His basic hypothesis was that cancer cells are fed by glucose (sugar). As a result, sugar has frequently been held responsible for the development of cancer. However, the ketogenic diet really takes advantage of the cancer's reliance on glucose. According to laboratory tests, at least some cancer cells have trouble utilising ketones as a fuel source. Due to biochemical modifications related to their capacity to utilise ketones, these cancer cells are less likely to undergo keto-adaptation.

According to the notion, the ketogenic diet gives healthy cells an advantage over malignant cells by purposefully inducing ketosis. That's because it's possible that cancer cells won't be as adept at utilising ketones for proliferation. Since keto reduces insulin levels in the body, it's theoretically plausible that it contributes to cancer. Research has shown that both insulin and growth factors like insulin can promote the development of tumors. New blood vessels must form to sustain the tumor for malignancies to continue to spread. Angiogenesis is the name of this process. It was discovered that keto reduces angiogenesis in a mouse model of the brain tumour glioma. Last but not least, it has been suggested that ketone bodies may directly harm cancer cells. In one study, researchers examined how additional ketone affected both mice with metastatic cancer and cancer cells generated in the lab. Ketone supplementation in the lab restricted the cancer cells' ability to survive and develop. According to the particular ketone body employed, more ketone was associated with 50–68% longer longevity in the cancer-bearing mice. Due to the rigorous nature of the keto diet, it may be challenging to obtain all the necessary nutrients for a balanced meal. Another issue might be the rise in fat consumption. For instance, some kinds of breast cancer have been associated with a lower chance of recurrence when eating a low-fat diet. However, because obesity is associated with a higher risk of breast cancer recurrence, it may help some people lose weight.

Your body might not operate as it does in cancer-free people if you are fighting with cancer or if you have an inherited disease of fat metabolism. It's likely that healthy cells experience issues processing the proteins and lipids, just as cancer cells may. Restriction of foods like fruits is a serious concern. Numerous studies have shown that persons who consume more fruits and vegetables have a lower risk of developing cancer. Since certain keto diets forbid dairy products, a deficiency in vitamin D might also be a problem. That being said, everyone with cancer should get a blood test to check their vitamin D level and speak to their oncologist if the level is low because low vitamin D levels have been linked to worse outcomes in some cancers (or within the low end of the normal range) Some ketogenic diets forbid dairy products, therefore a deficiency in vitamin D might be a problem. Poorer results in several malignancies are linked to low vitamin D levels. Every cancer patient should get their vitamin D level checked through a blood test, and if it is low, they should consult an oncologist.

Contraindications

Women who are pregnant, trying to get pregnant, or nursing should not follow the ketogenic diet. Additionally, those who have diabetes should only use it carefully and under a doctor's supervision. Keto should never be used to treat any of the following medical conditions. These conditions include;

A liver problem

Pancreatitis

A few inherited illnesses, including pyruvate kinase deficiency, and other metabolic abnormalities of fat.

Guidelines for Maintaining a Ketogenic Diet

The ketogenic diet is giving many individuals a secure, all-natural way to prevent and recover from cancer, which is on the rise. While the macronutrient ratios needed to enter ketosis vary depending on each person, a basic rule of thumb is to limit your daily carbohydrate intake to 50 grams. Healthy fats and moderate protein intake should account for the majority of calories. Here are a few simple ketogenic diet meal suggestions:

• Breakfast: avocado, pastured pork sausage, and eggs fried in grass-fed butter. For an additional burst of healthy fats, you might also add a tablespoon of coconut oil, avocado oil, fish oil, or MCT oil.

• Wild salmon over a sizable organic green salad dressed with extra virgin olive oil and Kalamata olives for lunch. Another choice would be burgers of pastured lamb with mint gremolata, olives, and greens (with oil or duck fat).

• Snack: Brazil nuts, macadamia nuts, grass-fed pemmican, or canned mackerel... another spoonful of your preferred healthy fat

• Dinner: Green salad with olive or avocado oil and free-range grilled duck legs (or duck confit) over mashed cauliflower. Another choice is grass-fed ribeye steak served with a ton of steamed vegetables and basil pesto. Before bed, add another spoonful of your preferred healthy fat.

Make sure you consume at least 8–10 servings of very low–carb, phytonutrient–rich vegetables (limitless amounts of organic kale, spinach, beet greens, with some organic cucumber, zucchini, and peppers), low—sugar berries (half a cup of organic raspberries or blackberries), and alkalizing lemon in addition to the suggestions mentioned above. A whole food juice is an easy method to increase your intake of these potent nutrients. We have greater options to treat cancer with the safe, natural food that our ancestors used because science shows that it is mostly a disease of the metabolism. As always, seek advice from your doctor before changing your diet.

Ketogenic Paleo Dinner Rolls

Ingredients

2 tablespoons Organic Psyllium Husk Powder

Four large pastured eggs

Nutiva Organic Coconut Flour, 8 tablespoons (70 g)

Grated finely 1 medium zucchini (160 g)

Avocado oil, 2 tablespoons

Organic apple cider vinegar, 2 tablespoons

1/4 cup filtered water

1 tablespoon dry basil

Non-aluminum baking powder, 3 teaspoons

1/2 teaspoon table salt

Instructions

1. Set the oven to 350°F. Butter a sheet pan.

2. Combine coconut flour, baking soda, herbs, sea salt, and psyllium husk powder in a big basin.

3. Combine the eggs, apple cider vinegar, avocado oil, water, and shredded zucchini in a medium bowl.

4. Combine thoroughly by adding the dry components to the wet ones and using an electric mixer on medium speed.

5. Grease your hands and make golfball-sized mounds of dough.

6. Gently roll and set on baking sheet. (I left mine round, but if you like, you can flatten them a little or shape them into mini rolls.)

7. Transfer to the oven and baste with avocado oil. Bake for 45 minutes or until golden brown and hollow when tapped, depending on size.

Information on Nutrition for Each Serving

74 calories, 2 g of saturated fat, 2 g of monounsaturated fat, 1 g of polyunsaturated fat, 2 g of NET carbohydrates, 0 g of sugar alcohols, 1 g of sugar, 3 g of fiber, 3 g of protein, 197 mg of potassium, 124 mg of phosphorous, 133 mg of sodium, and 6 mg of magnesium.

Sage- and cornbread-based paleo stuffing

You'll get the crunchy, golden goodness (and soft crumbly interior) of childhood Thanksgivings with this grain-free, gluten-free, Paleo stuffing. But this tasty meal is just only 7 carbs and 186 calories, compared to the roughly 400 calories and 44 carbs per serving of traditional stuffing. In addition to 7 grams of protein per serving

Add these ingredients for a hearty Sausage, Cranberry & "Cornbread" Stuffing: 1 cup of dried, organic, unsweetened cranberries and 1/2 pound of crumbled, sweet Italian turkey sausage

To the "Cornbread" Stuffing with Pear, Proscuitto, and 2 Bosc pears, diced when ripe but still firm, 4 ounces thinly sliced prosciutto, cut into ribbons, and 1/3 cup toasted chopped hazelnuts

Ingredients

• Ten big eggs

• 0.5 teaspoons of Celtic Sea Salt

• 10 tablespoons of melted grass-fed butter

• 1 big, chopped organic onion

• 1 chopped, entire organic leek

• 3 finely sliced organic celery ribs

• 2 Tsp. of dried thyme

• 2 teaspoons of dried sage

• 1/2 tsp. baking powder made without aluminum

• 2 minced garlic cloves

• 2 tablespoons minced fresh parsley

• 11 Tbsp. Organic Coconut Flour from Bob's Red Mill

Think about organic free-range chicken broth.

Instructions

1. Start by making the "cornbread." Set oven to 400 degrees Fahrenheit.

2. Combine the baking powder, salt, and coconut flour in a bowl.

3. Melt 1/2 cup of butter.

4. Beat eight eggs in an adequate basin. The melted butter is whisked in.

5. Combine the egg/butter combination with the coconut flour mixture by adding it and stirring.

6. Split the batter among 12 muffin tins that have been buttered. 25 minutes in the oven, or until golden brown. Allow to cool a bit.

Cut the corn muffins into cubes measuring 12 inch. On a cookie sheet coated with unbleached parchment paper, distribute the cubes and crumbs evenly in a single layer. Place in oven and dry and crisp for an hour at 250 degrees.

7. Set the oven's temperature to 400.

8. Over medium-high heat, melt the remaining 2 Tbsp. of butter in a big skillet. When the vegetables are tender and transparent, add the onion, leek, and celery. For about a minute, add the garlic, sage, and thyme. Add the parsley after taking the pan off the heat.

9. Butter a 13" x 9" pan. Combine the celery mixture with the muffin cubes and pan juices.

10. Combine the two remaining eggs with the chicken broth after beating them. Then bread mixture with the liquid. With your hands, gently blend the ingredients, being sure to coat the bread cubes in the liquid.

11. Place in the oven and bake, uncovered, for 45 to 1 hour, or until the top is crisp and brown.

Pancake made of buttermilk that burns fat (diary free, gluten free)

The weekends are the ideal time to splurge on breakfast. However, being "indulgent" need not be unhealthy! In truth, you can eat scrumptious breakfast dishes that will fill you up, keep your blood sugar steady, and keep your metabolism working at full capacity, like these Paleo buttermilk pancakes. But allow me to emphasize something crucial. The pancakes I'm referring to are vastly dissimilar from buttermilk pancakes. Additionally, they are much superior to "whole wheat" or even "organic" pancake mixes that you can buy in the supermarket. Whole wheat actually elevates blood sugar levels higher than almost any other food, even table sugar and candy bars!

And for your health, that is pretty bad news. High blood sugar levels cause inflammation and encourage the storage of abdominal fat. It raises the risk of diabetes, heart disease, fatty liver, and numerous other chronic ailments. The good news is that you can cook delectable breakfast meals that your entire family will enjoy without using a single grain. You will like feeding your family, too.

Benefits

• High protein content (12 g in each serving!)

• High in beneficial fats

• Low-glycemic, low-carb, and low-sugar

• No gluten

• Free of grains

• Non-Dairy

• No Soy

• No Corn

They are also a strong source of iron, vitamin B12, and phosphorus, as well as selenium, riboflavin, riboflavin, and fiber. So feel free to have a big stack of these filling breakfast snacks. Your health and taste buds will appreciate it!

Ingredients

- One-half cup coconut flour

- 1 tablespoon baking soda

- 2 teaspoons cinnamon

- Half a cup of coconut milk

- 6 pastured eggs

- 1 tbsp. Coconut Secret Coconut Nectar

- Sweet Leaf Stevia Clear Liquid Stevia, 8–10 drops (to taste)

Instructions

1. In a blender or mixer, thoroughly combine the coconut nectar, eggs, and coconut buttermilk.

2. Include the baking soda, cinnamon, and coconut flour. Blend until smooth

3. Give the batter five minutes to rest.

4. Set a secure nonstick griddle to medium heat; preferably one made of enameled cast iron. To prepare pancakes, pour batter into the pan (silver dollar-sized work best). About a minute on each side, then flip. Continually produce batches.

5. Top with a pat of Kerrygold Butter, my low-glycemic Antioxidant Super-Syrup, or a simple sauce made from organic frozen blueberries.

Drinks, beverages, and tonics

Cinnamon Hot Chocolate

Time to Prepare: 5 minutes

Cooking Period: 5 minutes

Serves four

Serving size: (without marshmallows) 5g fat (3g saturated), 37g carbohydrates, 3g fiber, 10g protein, and 129mg salt make up 217 calories.

The cinnamon sticks MUST be cooked in the milk mixture in order for this recipe to be suitable for individuals on the LMD (Low Microbial Diet).

Ingredients:

Cocoa powder, 1/4 cup

4 sticks of cinnamon (1 per mug)

2 ounces of semisweet chocolate, or about 13 cup,

Sugar, 1/4 cup

4 mugs of milk

Marshmallows, small (optional)

Cooking Guidelines:

1. In a saucepan, combine the chocolate, milk, and cocoa powder. Heat over medium-high heat. As the mixture boils and the chocolate melts, whisk continuously.

2. To add a hint of cinnamon taste, ladle the hot chocolate into glasses and stir with cinnamon sticks.

3. Add small marshmallows on the top of each mug to dress it up!

Recipes for Juicing

Fresh fruits and vegetables make the tastiest juices since they are nature's own containers for them. Fresh juice is packed with vitamins and phytochemicals that fight cancer in a form that the body can easily absorb.

Did you realize? The majority of the nutrients available in 5 cups of finely chopped carrot or celery are present in 1 cup of juice from those vegetables.

You'll need a juice extractor to start juicing.

• Department stores provide a variety of models ranging in price from $20 to $300 for individuals who don't already have one but are interested in purchasing one.

• If you frequently juice, high-tech features (such the capacity to handle whole, uncut fruits) are worth the extra cost. If not, a simple model will work.

Citrus juicers and juice extractors are the 2 sorts.

• Extractors are more adaptable; the majority of them contain a pulp collector that extracts the fiber, so you should still eat whole fruits and vegetables.

• Look for a machine with parts that can be easily cleaned or that can go in the dishwasher.

Make sure to read the instructions that came with your juicer so that you are familiar with how it operates and the recipes it includes. After each usage, make sure you thoroughly wash your juicer with hot, soapy water.

NOTE: People following the Low Microbial Diet SHOULD NOT make these recipes (LMD).

Apple and carrot juice

Ingredients:

3–4 medium-sized carrots

1 small Granny Smith apple

The sweetness of carrot juice contrasts favorably with the bitterness of the apples. Choose firm Granny Smiths when shopping for them because their juice will be clearer.

10 ounces include 200 calories, 0 fat, 49 carbohydrates, and 4 g of protein.

Juice of spinach, cucumber, and celery

Ingredients

2 cups packed spinach (4 oz.)

1 cucumber

1 stalk of celery

Celery doesn't overwhelm, so the spinach and cucumber juices can really shine. A good supply of calcium, iron, and potassium is spinach.

10 ounces provide 139 calories, 1 g of fat, 35 g of carbohydrates, and 1 g of protein.

Blueberry, pineapple, and ginger juice

Ingredients

1/4 pineapple

1 cup of Blueberries

1 slice (1/4-1/2 inch) of fresh ginger

Antioxidants, which have been demonstrated to help fight several types of cancer, are abundant in blueberries. When mixed with pineapple, ginger promotes digestion and creates a South Pacific atmosphere.

80 calories, 0 fat grams, 16 carbohydrates, and 7g of protein are in 12 ounces.

Avoid berries and pick a fruit that doesn't contain berries for LMD.

Eggnog

Salmonella is not a concern with this dish because it has been cooked. You have a choice between the full high-fat version and the reduced-fat version. Please consult your doctor before adding alcohol because it is hard on your liver, just like chemotherapy medications are.

12 (1-half cup servings)

Serving size: (Low fat version) 135 calories, 2g of saturated fat, 2g of total fat, 5g of protein, 120mg of sodium, 18g of carbohydrates, 0g of fiber, and 46mg of cholesterol.

NOTE: Avoid alcohol for LMD. Select lactose-free milk for a diet that is lactose-free. Alternatives include substituting an extract for the alcohol and Lactaid milk for ordinary milk.

Ingredients:

6 glasses of nonfat milk

2 big eggs

All-purpose flour, 2 tablespoons

1 teaspoon vanilla extract

14 cup brandy, bourbon, or rum, or 2 teaspoons (or to taste) of rum or brandy extract

1/8 tbsp. freshly grated nutmeg

2/3 cups sugar

1/4 tsp. salt

Light whipping cream, 1/4 cup

(Optional) Cinnamon ground for garnish

Cooking Guidelines:

1. Over low heat, whisk occasionally, bring milk and nutmeg to a simmer in a heavy medium saucepan.

2. Blend the eggs, sugar, flour, and salt in a sizable basin. Return the mixture to the pot while adding the hot milk gradually while whisking.

3. Cook eggnog over a very low heat, continually stirring, for 10 to 15 minutes, or until it is thick enough to coat the back of a spoon. (Eggnog must be heated to 160°F; do not allow it to simmer.) Remove from heat and pour into a basin after passing through a fine-mesh strainer.

4. Stir in the extracts. The eggnog should be covered with plastic wrap and placed in the refrigerator for at least 8 hours or overnight to chill. (The eggnog can be kept in the fridge for up to two days if it is covered.)

5. Add cream to eggnog right before serving. Pour into cups and top with additional freshly grated cinnamon or nutmeg.

Hot Healthy Winter Teas

Flavored chai

Serves four

74 calories, 1g fat, 16g carbohydrates, 2g protein, 0g fiber, and 27mg sodium per serving.

Ingredients:

4 pods of green cardamom

4 complete cloves

1-stick of cinnamon

3 pieces of thinly sliced ginger

One cup of nonfat milk (for lactose-free diet, choose lactose-free milk)

4-6 Whole black peppercorns

3 cups of water

3 tbsp. of brown sugar or honey

1-2 bags of black tea, either regular or decaf.

Cooking Guidelines:

Place cardamom, cloves, cinnamon, ginger, peppercorns, and water in a big saucepan. Heating to a boil Low-heat simmering for five minutes. Turn off heat. 15 minutes of steeping under cover. Add honey or brown sugar and milk. Reheat to a simmer. Turn off heat. Depending on the desired strength of tea, add the tea bags and let them steep for 2–5 minutes. Serve heated after straining. (Be sure to add the ground dried spices at the end and not during cooking if you choose to use them in place of the entire spices specified above. Otherwise, they'll ruin the consistency of the chai.)

Flavored green tea

Serves four

140 calories, 0g fat, 33g carbohydrates, 1g protein, 0g fiber, and 35mg sodium per serving.

Ingredients:

1 stick of cinnamon

4 complete cloves

4 cups of natural, unsweetened cherry juice (for LMD choose pasteurized cherry juice)

4 star nutmeg

3–4 green tea bags, with the option of decaf

Cooking Guidelines:

Over a medium heat, boil cherry juice. spice up. For an additional five minutes, simmer on a lower heat if necessary. Cut the heat off. For 10 minutes, cover and let the spices seep in the juice. Tea bags should be added and steeped for 2 to 5 minutes, depending on the desired strength. Serve heated after straining.

Ginger, lemon, and honey in the Chamomile-Mint Soother

Serves four

1 g or less of all nutrients per serving.

Ingredients:

3 cups of water

1 tablespoon fresh ginger root, minced

Lemon and honey, to taste (for LMD, eliminate honey and choose another sweetener)

3-tablespoon chamomile tea

1Tbsp. of dried mint

Cooking Guidelines:

Bring water and ginger to a boil in a big pot. Reduce heat, and then simmer for five minutes. Include mint and chamomile. Steep for 10 minutes with the lid on. Add honey and lemon to taste after straining.

Rosemary and Celery Tonic

It's a good thing that cool, herbal, vegetable-infused beverages are popular right now. Simple drinks made with vegetable purée are a terrific way to stay hydrated and obtain your recommended daily allowance of vegetables. With celery, lemon juice, and rosemary, this nutritious tonic creates a cool, green beverage with just a hint of heat from the cayenne. It is a healthy beverage that you can feel good about consuming even with the slightest amount of sweetness. What's not to love about the ingredients, which also give you fiber, antioxidants, vitamins, and minerals? For breakfast, a special dinner, or during a barbecue, combine it in a blender and pour it over ice.

Ingredients

• Two medium celery stalks with leaves, cut into quarters

• Half a teaspoon of fresh rosemary

• One little lemon, juiced (about 2 tbsp)

- A teaspoon of agave nectar

- Add a pinch of cayenne pepper

- Use pinch salt

- 1 cup of water

- Cubes of ice

It yields two servings. 20 calories, 0 g total fat (0 g saturated fat, 0 g trans-fat), 0 mg of cholesterol, 5 g of carbs, 0 g of protein, 1 g of dietary fiber, 180 mg of sodium, 4 g of sugar, and 3 g of added sugar are all contained in one serving.

Directions

1. Fill the container of a powerful blender with the celery, rosemary, lemon juice, agave nectar, cayenne pepper, salt, and water.

2. Process the mixture for a few minutes, or until it is thoroughly liquefied.

3. Pour the celery combination into each of the two glasses after adding ice to each.

Notes

Fresh rosemary can be replaced with dried rosemary.

Agave nectar can be swapped out for pure maple syrup.

A pinch is roughly equal to 1/8 teaspoon.

Orange Rhubarb Refresher

Enjoy this special blend of rhubarb, orange, and mint to cool off and celebrate the summer. In addition to vitamin C, lutein and zeaxanthin, two phytochemicals with antioxidant characteristics that belong to the carotenoid family, are present in one glass.

Ingredients

• 3/4 lb. of 3 cups fresh rhubarb, sliced crosswise into 1/2-inch slices.

• Four cups of cold water

• One cup of cut strawberries

• 1 glass of orange juice

• 4 garnishing mint sprigs

Has eight servings (about 3.5 oz per serving). 30 calories, 0 g total fat (including 0 g of saturated fat and 0 g of trans fat), 0 mg cholesterol, 7 g of carbs, 1 g of protein, 1 g of dietary fiber, 0 mg of sodium, 4 g of sugar, and 0 g of added sugar are included in each serving.

Directions

1. Combine the rhubarb and water in a sizable non-reactive saucepan made of stainless steel or another material. Over medium-high heat, cover and bring to a boil.

2. Lower the temperature, then simmer for 15 minutes. Ten minutes of steeping are recommended for the covered pot.

3. Place the big strainer on top of the bowl. Fill the strainer with the pot's contents, then pour the liquid into the bowl. Press the rhubarb very softly with the back of a wooden spoon to draw out any juice that drains easily. If you press too hard, the infusion will get hazy. Throw away pulp.

4. Pour the liquid, which should be about 4 cups, into a glass jar or other container and allow it to come to room temperature before covering it and storing it in the refrigerator for up to 2 days.

5. Measure 3 cups of rhubarb infusion to be used in Refresher. Pour 1/2 cup into a pitcher, then stir in the

strawberries. Add the remaining orange juice and rhubarb infusion.

6. Distribute Refresher among four tall glasses filled with ice. If used, place a mint sprig on top of each glass.

7. To make a single serving, combine 1/4 cup rhubarb infusion with 2 strawberries in a glass. To the remaining 1/2 cup infusion, 1/4 cup orange juice, and ice, add a splash of cold water.

Pink Ginger Lemonade

Tart lemonade softened with red berries, which give it a gorgeous pink hue and a sweet flavor, mixes wonderfully with the spiciness and sweetness of ginger. The berries provide the majority of the natural sweetness to balance the lemons in this thirst-quenching beverage, which is as gorgeous as it is tasty, with only a small amount of agave nectar. During the week, keep it in the fridge as a healthy hydration alternative. Serve it over ice in pitchers at gatherings.

Ingredients

- 2 1/2 glasses of water

- 1 inch of freshly peeled ginger

- 2 tablespoons agave nectar

- One-third cup of cut strawberries or raspberries (fresh or frozen)

- Freshly squeezed lemon juice in 3/4 cup (6 medium lemons)

Contains 4 servings (1 cup). 50 calories, 0 g of total fat (0 g saturated, 0 g trans), 0 mg of cholesterol, 13 g of carbs, 0 g of protein, 1 g of dietary fiber, 0 mg of sodium, 10 g of sugar, and 8 g of added sugar are all contained in one serving.

Directions

1. Fill the blender container with water, ginger, agave nectar, berries, and lemon juice.

2. Continue processing until the mixture is smooth.

3. Convert to a pitcher and keep chilled until ready to serve. Serve chilled.

Notes

*You can use honey or maple syrup instead.

Water melon granita

This dessert is a straightforward adaptation of a summertime favorite. Lycopene, a strong antioxidant, and vitamins C and A are all present in watermelon. Prepare this delicacy for your upcoming summer party or whenever you're in the mood for something tasty and cool.

Ingredients

- 2 limes

- 2 teaspoons divided sugar

- 1/3 water

- Cubes of 1 1/2 to 2 pounds seedless watermelon

- Mint leaves, if preferred, as a garnish

Approximately 3/4 cup each serving; yields 4 servings. Each serving contains 70 calories, 0 grams of total fat (0 g of saturated fat, 0 g of trans fat), 0 mg of cholesterol, 19 grams of carbohydrates, 1 g of protein, 1 g of dietary fiber, 0 mg of sodium, 15 grams of sugar, and 2 grams of added sugar.

Directions

1. using a fine grater, remove the limes' exterior green layer (the "zest"). Combine the zest, 1 teaspoon of sugar, and 1/4 cup of lime juice in a small bowl. 1/3 cup water and the remaining sugar should be combined in a small saucepan. Boil the mixture. Add zest mixture once sugar has dissolved. Stir after removing from heat, and then allow it cool to room temperature.

2. Puree the melon in a blender or food processor to yield 3 cups of liquid. Place in a metal 9" × 9" pan. Mix in the syrup. Place in the freezer, then wrap with plastic. After 6 to 8 hours of freezing, stir. Scrape well with a fork and scoop into serving bowls before serving.

3. If preferred, garnish with mint and serve right away.

Hot cider with ginger and turmeric

A warm cup of apple cider is the ideal wintertime beverage. This version includes the two powerful spices, ginger and turmeric, for a particular flavor and nutritional profile. For instance, fresh ginger includes a spicy component called gingerol, while turmeric gets its distinctive yellow color from the group of compounds known as curcuminoids that fight cancer. Both are being investigated for their antioxidant and anti-inflammatory capacities.

Ingredients

- One cup of delicious, fresh apple cider

- 1 teaspoon freshly grated ginger

- 1 teaspoon freshly grated turmeric

- 1 strip of lemon peel, white part included, measuring 1/2 inch by 1/2 inch.

- An optional dash of cinnamon

Produces 1 serving (1 cup). 130 calories, 0 g of total fat (0 g saturated, 0 g trans), 0 mg of cholesterol, 31 g of carbs, 0 g of protein, 1 g of dietary fiber, 25 mg of sodium, and 26 g of sugar are all contained in one serving.

Directions:

1. Combine cider, ginger, turmeric, and lemon peel in a small saucepan. Heat for 3 minutes over medium-high heat, or until a ring of bubbles forms around the pan's edge.

2. Cover the pan and leave it for 5 minutes to steep.

3. Add a dash of cinnamon, if desired, and strain the hot spiced cider through a fine tea strainer into a mug. Serve right away.

Responsiveness of the body to cancer and treatments

According to research, exercise is generally safe and beneficial before, during, and after cancer therapy. It can enhance your quality of life and give you more energy to do the activities you enjoy. Exercise may also lessen your risk of developing new cancers in the future and assist you in coping with treatment-related adverse effects. Spending too much time lying down or sitting still can lead to decreased range of motion, muscle weakening, and loss of physical function. Many cancer care teams advise their patients to stay as physically active as possible before, during, and after cancer treatment. How staying active can benefit you before, during, and after treatment for cancer

• Facilitate improved brain and body function

• Tiredness (fatigue)

• Promote depression and anxiety reduction

- May improve your quality of sleep

- Maintain or enhance your physical stamina for work

- Increase your range of motion, bone density, and muscle strength.

- Boost your immune system.

- Increases your appetite

- Assist you in achieving and keeping a healthy weight

- Might be beneficial for lymphedema brought on by breast cancer (and does not increase risk)

- Reduce the likelihood that some cancers may recur.

- Enhance your standard of living

- lessen side effects of medication

Chapter 4

Physical and clinical approach to cancer treatment

•After diagnosis and therapy, avoid idleness and resume your regular daily activities as soon as you can.

• Engage in consistent physical activity.

• Increase your level of physical exercise gradually at first.

• Increase your weekly activity to 150–300 minutes of moderate activity (or 75–150 minutes of vigorous activity).

•Work out for at least 10 minutes at a time, multiple times per week.

•Include at least two days a week of resistance training activity.

•Stretch out at least twice a week.

The aims of a workout regimen
Before therapy.

Before therapy, increasing your level of physical activity or maintaining it may make it easier for you to handle and recover from the treatment. According to research, being as active as you can while undergoing surgery may help you heal more quickly. Additionally, once you start treatment, exercise may provide you more energy, a better night's sleep, and a better ability to deal with stress and worry. Many people discover that it may be more difficult to be active once their treatment program has begun. Therefore, having better physical condition at the beginning means you can handle greater activities both during and after treatment.

During therapy

Your capacity to exercise while receiving therapy may be impacted by certain factors, such as:

• The nature and stage of your cancer

• Your chemotherapy

• Your degree of strength, endurance, and fitness both before and after therapy

You might need to exercise less or at a lower intensity during treatment if you exercised before. To remain as active as you can is the objective. People undergoing cancer treatment who were very sedentary may need to begin with brief, low-intensity exercise, such as quick walks. If there are any restrictions on what you can do when exercising during treatment, discuss them with your cancer care team.

After therapy

The majority of people can gradually increase their exercise duration and intensity as their negative effects subside. For some cancer survivors, an activity that could be low-or moderate-intensity for a healthy person may appear like a high-intensity activity. As you steadily increase your activity, take your time and be kind to yourself. The most crucial thing to keep in mind is to move as much as you can.

Physical activity is crucial to your general health and quality of life at this time. According to research, maintaining a healthy weight, eating healthily, and exercising may help lower the risk of developing secondary cancer as well as other dangerous chronic conditions. If you have osteoporosis, cancer that has metastasized to the bone, arthritis, nerve damage, poor vision, poor balance, or weakness; avoid using heavy weights or performing workouts that place too much stress on your bones. You can have a higher chance of getting harmed or breaking a bone.

Keep exercising simple and enjoyable.

Each person has a different ideal level of exercise. The ideal level of activity for someone with cancer is unknown. Your exercise regimen should assist you maintain your muscle strength and your ability to perform the tasks you need and wish to perform. You'll be able to exercise and perform better the more active you are. Even so, it's still advisable to continue staying active as much as you can by continuing to engage in your regular activities. The secret to remaining active is to keep your fitness routine straightforward and enjoyable. The best strategies to reduce stress are through exercise and relaxation methods. Getting better and maintaining good health both depend on reducing stress.

Tips for maintaining your exercise regimen

• Create both immediate and long-term goals.

• Keep the fun in mind.

• Make a change to keep it interesting. Try tai chi, yoga, or dancing.

• Recruit friends, family, and coworkers to join you in your workout regimen.

Use charts or a fitness tracker to keep track of your activity progress.

• Acknowledge and honor your accomplishments.

Even for someone in good health, beginning an exercise regimen can be challenging. If you suffer from a chronic disease, it could be even more difficult, especially if you weren't used to working out before your diagnosis. Slowly start out and work your way up. If you were an avid exerciser before receiving a cancer diagnosis, you might need to temporarily lower the intensity and duration of your workouts. However, you can build back up when you're ready.

Include exercise in your everyday regimen.

There are methods to incorporate physical activity into your daily routine. Do only what you feel capable of doing, always.

• Go for a stroll after dinner.

• Ride a bicycle.

- Rake the leaves rather than using a blower to cut the grass.

- Clean up your bathroom.

- Wax and clean your vehicle

- Play activities that require physical activity with children, such as jump rope, freeze tag, and other games you enjoyed as a child.

- Take a controlled dog on a walk so that you don't trip or lose your balance.

- Clean up the garden.

- Dance around in your living room.

- While watching TV, use a treadmill or exercise bike, or perform crunches, squats, lunges, and arm curls.

- Stroll to lunch

- Leave your vehicle in the farthest available parking space at work, and then stroll inside.

- Take the stairs rather than the escalator or elevator.

- Exit the bus a few stops early and continue walking.

• Schedule 10-minute walking breaks for yourself in your daily planner.

• Create a walking club with your coworkers to keep you inspired to walk throughout the workday.

• Try using a fitness tracker to do more steps each day.

Cancer patients may need to exercise less vigorously and build up their fitness program more slowly than non-cancer patients. Keep in mind that the objective is to be as active as you can. Make it interesting, safe, and useful for you by maintaining all three.

Color ribbons and cancer

Many people don ribbons to support loved ones who are battling cancer and to raise awareness of that particular type of disease. The ribbon colors are chosen by nationally renowned non-profit groups that offer support, information, and awareness for each of the various illnesses. Different colors stand for various types of cancer. There are also other formally acknowledged annual cancer awareness months.

The following table includes the most prevalent cancer kinds, the ribbon colors that correspond to each type, and the awareness months for each cancer.

Color Chart for Cancer Ribbons

Color Chart for Cancer Ribbons	
CELEBRATION MONTH	
National Cancer Prevention Month February	
National Minority Cancer Awareness Month	April
National Young Adult Cancer Awareness Week April 1-7	
National Cancer Research Month	May
Oncology Nursing Month	May
Cancer Immunotherapy Awareness Month	June
Cancer Survivors Month June	
National Black Family Cancer Awareness Week June 17-23	
CELEBRATION &MONTH	COLOUR
All cancers	Lavender
Appendix cancer None	Amber
Bladder cancer May	Marigold/blue/purple

Brain cancer May	Gray
Breast cancer October	Pink
Cervical cancer January	Teal/white
Childhood cancer September	Gold
Colon cancer March	Dark blue
Esophageal cancer April	Periwinkle
Gallbladder cancer February	Kelly green
Head and neck cancer April	Burgundy/ivory
Hodgkin's lymphoma September	Violet
Kidney cancer March	Orange
Leiomyosarcoma July	Purple
Leukemia September	Orange
Liver cancer October	Emerald
Lung cancer November	White
Lymphoma	Lime green

September		
Melanoma and skin cancers May	Black	
Multiple myeloma March	Burgundy	
Ovarian cancer September	Teal	
Pancreatic cancer November	Purple	
Prostate cancer September	Light blue	
Sarcoma/bone cancer July	Yellow	
Stomach/gastric cancer November	Periwinkle	
Testicular cancer April	Orchid	
Thyroid cancer September	Teal/pink/blue	
Uterine cancer September	Peach	
Neuroendocrine/carcinoid cancer November	Zebra stripe	
Honors caregivers November	Plum	

The table includes; the most prevalent cancer kinds, the ribbon colors that correspond to each type, and the awareness months for each cancer.

Clinical treatment for cancer

The course of treatment varies greatly depending on the type and stage of the cancer as well as the patient's general condition. Chemotherapy, radiation therapy, and surgery are the most widely used treatments. Other treatments include cryosurgery, photodynamic therapy, angiogenesis inhibitors, hematopoietic stem cell transplants, targeted/biological therapies, and angiogenesis inhibitors. There are potential dangers, advantages, and side effects with every treatment. The best and most suitable course of therapy will be decided by the patient and members of their care team, which may include an internist or other specialist, a surgeon, an oncologist, a radiation oncologist, and others.

There is still no cure for cancer, despite significant investment and effort. Known as the "National Cancer Moonshot" by President Barack Obama, the United States stated in 2016 that it will invest $1 billion in the search for such a treatment. The best method to prevent cancer is through a healthy lifestyle, at least until a cure is discovered. Eating lots of fruits and vegetables, keeping a healthy weight, quitting smoking, using alcohol sparingly, exercising, avoiding sun damage, being immunized, and having routine health tests are a few strategies to help prevent cancer.

Surgery

Malignant tumors are frequently removed with surgery. Surgery enables the precise measurement of the tumor's size as well as the degree of invasion and spread to neighboring tissues or lymph nodes, all crucial elements in the prognosis and management of the condition. Chemotherapy and/or radiation therapy are frequently used in conjunction with surgery as a cancer treatment. Sometimes it is impossible to completely eliminate cancer surgically due to the risk of damaging vital organs or tissues. DE bulking surgery is used in this situation to get rid of as much of the tumor as is safe. Similar to this, palliative surgery is done in cases of advanced cancer to lessen the consequences of a cancerous tumor (such as pain or discomfort). DE bulking and palliative operations aim to lessen the consequences of the malignancy but are not curative. After cancer surgery, reconstructive surgery can be used to improve the appearance or functionality of a bodily part. An illustration of this kind of surgery is breast reconstruction following a mastectomy.

Radiation treatment

A widely popular cancer treatment is radiation. Radiation therapy is given to patients with cancer in around half of all cases; it may be given prior to, during, or following chemotherapy and/or surgery. Radiation can be given internally or externally, with the latter including the delivery of X-rays, gamma rays, or other high-energy particles to the affected area from outside the body. Placing radioactive material within the body close to cancer cells is known as internal radiation therapy. The term for this is brachytherapy. The oral or intravenous injection of radioactive medicine results in systemic radiation. The malignant tissue is directly reached by the radioactive substance. Systemic radiation therapies include radioactive iodine (I-131 for thyroid cancer) and strontium-89 (for bone cancer).

External radiation is typically administered over a period of 5 to 8 weeks, 5 days a week. Sometimes, different treatment plans are applied.

Chemotherapy Technique

Chemotherapy, also known as "chemo," is the name given to more than 100 distinct drugs that are used to treat cancer and other diseases. If eradicating all cancer cells is not achievable, treatment objectives can instead include symptom relief, slowing the growth of the cancer, and preventing it from spreading (such as pain).

The drugs may be administered orally, intravenously (IV), intramuscularly (IM), topically, or via injection depending on the form of chemotherapy recommended. A catheter or port, which is typically implanted in a chest blood vessel for the length of the therapy, may be used to administer IV chemotherapy. Regional chemotherapy can occasionally be provided right to the place that requires it. In the case of treating bladder cancer, intravesical therapy involves injecting chemotherapy right into the bladder. The type and stage of the cancer, any prior cancer treatment, and the patient's general health all influence the chemotherapy regimen that is given to a patient. Chemotherapy is typically given in cycles over the course of a few days, a few weeks, or several months, with rest intervals in between.

Other Therapies

Other therapies, in addition to surgery, radiation therapy, and chemotherapy, are employed to treat cancer. These consist of:

Biological or targeted therapies

Targeted or biological therapies aim to combat cancer and strengthen the body's defenses while causing the least amount of harm to healthy, normal cells. Vaccines, cytokines, monoclonal antibodies, and immunomodulation medications are a few examples of targeted or biological therapy.

Transplants of hematopoietic stem cells

Hematopoietic stem cell transplants entail injecting stem cells into a cancer patient after high-dose chemotherapy and/or radiation have destroyed the bone marrow.

Inhibitors of Angiogenesis

Drugs called angiogenesis inhibitors prevent the development of new blood vessels, which malignant tumors require to grow.

Cryosurgery

Cryosurgery uses extremely freezing temperatures to destroy malignant and precancerous cells.

Photodynamic Treatment

A medicine known as a photosensitizing agent is used in photodynamic therapy (PDT) to make malignant cells sensitive to laser treatment. PDT involves the application of laser light of a specific wavelength to tissue. Photodynamic therapy selectively kills cancer cells while

causing the least amount of harm to neighboring
healthy, normal tissues.

Chapter 5

Surviving cancer

From the moment of diagnosis forward, a person is referred to as a "cancer survivor." The word "survivor" connotes strength and positivity to many individuals. Others don't like labels and would rather look ahead to a time when cancer is not the main concern. According to research, learning what to anticipate after completing primary cancer treatment can help you get ready for life after cancer. The survivorship phase is recognized as this.

Survivorship care tries to maintain your mental and physical health after primary cancer treatment is over. This might involve support for managing adverse effects of treatment and continuing a healthy lifestyle following treatment.

Establishing a new standard

You might anticipate that once therapy is over, things will soon get back to normal. Alternately, you might view the diagnosis as a chance to improve your life. Cancer survivors frequently develop a new way of life over time. Finding a new normal phase is used to describe this process, and it might take months or even years to achieve it.

Recognizing your emotions

While the majority of people adjust to life after cancer treatment successfully over time, many people continue to harbor worries or fears. It can be possible for you to process your feelings if you acknowledge how you are feeling. It could be beneficial to think back on how you have handled challenging circumstances in the past to get some ideas for effective coping mechanisms. Most cancer survivors discover that their symptoms do improve with time.

Common responses to treatment completion

• Relief - You may feel relieved that the treatment is over and appears to have worked. The opportunity to concentrate on your interests may be welcomed by you.

• Isolation - When frequent appointments are fewer or stop altogether, you could feel anxious or lost. It could feel like you've lost your safety net. If your connections have altered or people don't comprehend what you've been through, you could also feel lonely.

• Fear — you can be afraid that the cancer will return.

• Uncertainty - If you are unsure about your health, you could put off making future plans. Although this is incredibly difficult, you can learn to handle it successfully.

• Frustration - You can feel frustrated if you believe that your loved ones are expecting too much of you. Or perhaps you feel defeated because you are unable to accomplish your goals.

• Optimistic - You might feel optimistic about the future and relieved to be returning to your regular routine.

• Survivor guilt: You could feel bad or wonder why you managed to beat cancer while others didn't. This may be upsetting.

• Anxiety - you can experience anxiety before to follow-up appointments or while anticipating test results.

• Worry - You can worry about the adverse effects of the treatment, how long they'll last, and whether they'll have an impact on your life. Numerous survivors are concerned about their financial situation or about burdening their families. Others fret about going back to work and handling inquiries from coworkers.

• Lack of confidence - you may have conflicting feelings about your appearance and wellbeing. You might not trust your body because you believe it has failed you, or you might be concerned about how it will affect your memory and cognitive function. Many people experience vulnerability and self-consciousness related to their sexuality and body image.

• Intensified feelings - You can cry or get emotional extremely quickly, especially when someone asks how you are. It is typical to experience this.

• Anger - You could feel furious about your cancer diagnosis and the way it has changed your life.

• Delayed feelings - now that therapy is done, you might discover that your emotions finally catch up with you. Many folks find this confusing because they don't anticipate having negative feelings when their treatment is over.

Retaining Hope

Your family and friends can tell you to "think positively." Being upbeat all the time is practically difficult because everyone experiences good and terrible days, both before and after receiving a cancer diagnosis. However, a lot of survivors claim that having hope made it easier for them to deal with their sickness and implement healthy lifestyle changes, such increasing their exercise or altering their nutrition.

After treatment is over, it's normal to feel down or melancholy. Even years after treatment, cancer survivors may face spells of concern or depression. You might experience sadness due to the changes that cancer has brought about, worry about the future, or dread of the illness returning. Many patients have a sense of separation from their pre-cancer lives. Others worry about their ability to find employment again and how their family will fare if they are unable to make ends meet. You might have low moods occasionally with no apparent cause.

You may find it easier to manage difficult times with the support of your loved ones, other cancer survivors, or medical professionals.

Controlling your emotions

• Look after yourself. Eat a balanced diet, get lots of water, and don't overindulge in alcohol.

• Engage in regular exercise. Anger, tension, anxiety, and sadness may all be managed, and sleep quality can be improved. A quick daily stroll will be beneficial.

• Establish connections with others who share your interests.

• Get close to a pet.

• Talk to a loved one about your worries and fears. You may feel less isolated as a result.

• Spend time outdoors, breathing clean air. Perhaps a change of scenery can make you feel better.

• Make a list of the things you'd like to do, and schedule time to do one of them every day.

• You can express yourself through writing, painting, coloring, music, or singing.

• Create a routine. Wake up at the same hour every day. Attempt to take a shower and dress.

• Occasionally, give yourself permission to have a "bad mood day." You don't need to be "up" all the time.

• Work on not being sucked into your ideas as they come and go. Attempt to avoid stressing about forthcoming exams or examinations and instead try to concentrate on the here and now.

• Keep a journal of the good things that occur every day. These things don't have to be significant; they could simply be a supportive grin from a neighbor.

Fear of a relapse of cancer

It's common to experience anxiety or fear that the cancer will return (recurrence). This worry will probably be felt to some extent by the majority of cancer survivors, and it may come and go for many years. You can develop coping mechanisms for this phobia. Your physical health, as well as your capacity to enjoy life and make plans for the future, may be impacted by worry about recurrence. Some survivors say it has cast a shadow or a gloomy cloud over their lives. This dread normally vanishes with time, although it occasionally comes back, for example:

• Before to examinations, exams, and scans

• Unique events, such birthdays or holidays

• The dates you were diagnosed, underwent surgery, or concluded your treatment;

• When further cancer patients are identified

• If you experience symptoms that were present at the time of your initial diagnosis

• The passing of a friend or relative

• stopping by the medical facility where you had treatment or going to see a friend there

• reading news articles on cancer, new treatments, and cancer patients in celebrity

• seeing marketing or fundraising efforts for cancer.

Signs for a new cancer growth

It's critical to understand your own sense of normalcy. Consult your General Practitioner as soon as you can if you detect any strange changes in your body or if you have any concerns. Don't wait until your upcoming appointment for a checkup.

The following are the primary warning signs and symptoms:

•An unhealed lump, sore, or ulcer

• A mole that bleeds or has altered in size, color, or shape

• A persistent cough, hoarseness, or a cough that produces blood

• A modification in bowel patterns, such as blood in feces, prolonged diarrhea, or constipation lasting longer than a week

• Issues or modifications with urination

• Chronic heartburn or swallowing issues

• Unusual bruising or bleeding

• Atypical modifications to the testicles or breasts

• Persistent abdominal (belly) pain or bloating

• Inexplicable changes in your general health, like weight gain or loss, sweating at night, a loss of appetite, or a lack of energy (fatigue).

In order to detect cancer in people before any symptoms arise, screening is organized testing. Australia has free nationwide screening programs for cervical cancer, breast cancer, and bowel cancer for persons aged 50 to 74. (Women aged 25–74). These are the only cancers for which organized screening has been shown beneficial at this time.

Ways to control fear of reoccurrence

• Discuss your risk of recurrence and how this will be handled with your treatment team. Ask about warning signs to look for and how to tell the difference between common aches, pains, and illnesses and cancer symptoms.

• Put your attention on the things you can control, such being present at your follow-up meetings and implementing lifestyle changes that will lower your chance of recurrence.

• Be aware of the symptoms of stress and worry, such as a racing heart or trouble sleeping. Manage them in a healthy way by practicing yoga, taking calm, deep breaths, or taking a walk, for example.

• Consult a counselor or psychologist if you have a severe fear of recurrence. They might be able to give you some tips on how to cope with your concerns. Consider joining a support group.

• Take into account engaging in a creative endeavor like writing, painting, or drawing. This helps some people process their feelings, according to them.

• Discuss with your doctor how to handle any side effects from continuous treatment, as they can make it more difficult to deal emotionally.

Work modification after chemotherapy

It's possible that you were able to take time from work to receive therapy. Now that your therapy is complete, you may be considering returning to your job. You could discover that returning to work aids in maintaining your sense of identity and social fit. Along with increasing your income, it might even make you feel better about yourself. Your job may serve as a reminder that you have a life outside of cancer. You are a cherished employee, a fantastic supervisor, or a dependable colleague. When you return to work, you'll also be in regular contact with other people. Being with people may be a huge comfort when dealing with cancer, which can often make you feel incredibly alone and isolated. If you're considering returning to the workforce, make sure your doctor has given you the all-clear first. You could also want to discuss with your employer the possibility of flextime, job sharing, telecommuting (working from home), or other solutions that could ease the transition back into the demands of your position. While some people may find it simple to make the switch to a full-time job, others may need some time to acclimate. At first, you could discover that you become tired easily or have problems focusing. Take care of yourself when you return to your "regular" life, and try to be patient.

Informing colleagues of your cancer treatment

It's up to you how honest you want to be with your coworkers about your health throughout and after cancer treatment. You can choose if and how much information you want to provide based on your relationships with your coworkers. Try not to feel compelled to explain or disclose things. Only you know what will work best for you and your circumstances. When you return to work, you could notice that your coworkers are responding to you in different ways. Your cancer diagnosis and absences may be met with sympathy and offers of assistance from people who understand what you've been going through. People may feel uneasy around you. Some people might be brought back to memories of a loved one's battle with cancer. Some coworkers could be irritated about having to take on more responsibilities on days when you weren't there. Others can avoid you altogether or obtrusively inquire about your health or the reason you haven't been around. It also helps to plan out how you will respond to other people's emotions and how much information you want to share in advance.

Legal safeguards for cancer patients

Regardless of whether you disclose your disease to coworkers or not, you are entitled to the same rights and opportunities as everyone else. Your abilities and credentials should be the sole determining factors in your employment, promotion, and treatment at work. You cannot be dismissed for being ill as long as you are capable of performing your job responsibilities. Additionally, you shouldn't be forced to take a job you would never have considered before your sickness.

Federal legislation like the Americans with Disabilities Act and the Rehabilitation Act safeguard many people with cancer-related employment issues (ADA). The Family and Medical Leave Act (FMLA), which allows many persons with serious diseases to take reasonable unpaid leave to receive medical attention or manage their symptoms, has further advantages for some people. To learn more about your alternatives, speak with a member of your human resources team or another professional with knowledge of the workplace. Resuming a regular work schedule may require some time for adjustment and additional assistance for certain persons. Your work may suffer if you attempt to resume a full-time schedule before you are prepared. As you choose how to return to the workforce, discuss your type of employment and any issues you are experiencing with your healthcare physician. Until you know how things turn out, you might need to start with shorter workdays or work fewer days per week. You might discover that your working style has altered or that you want additional assistance to complete your tasks.

Workplace modification

Employers are not compelled to offer personal-use equipment like spectacles or hearing aids or to decrease standards in order to accommodate an employee. However, unless the employer can demonstrate that doing so would place an unreasonable burden on them, they are required to make reasonable accommodations for qualifying disabled applicants or employees. The following are just a few examples of acceptable accommodations for cancer patients:

- Creating or altering tools or equipment

- Reorganizing a position

- Providing a flexible work schedule or the option to work from home, if possible.

• If an employee can no longer perform their current work, reassigning them to a position that is open or giving them new tasks.

• Modifying or adjusting exams, instruction manuals, or rules

• Improving accessibility and usability for individuals with impairments in the workplace

A counselor for vocational rehabilitation can assist you with some of your legal concerns regarding your employment, but you may also want to research laws that apply to you and how you can handle any issues that may arise. Ask your medical staff if any cancer treatment facilities offer recommendations to counselors in vocational rehabilitation. You might be able to get assistance from your medical team's resources or personnel.

Handling discrimination in workplace

Even if the general public's understanding of cancer is improving, there are still prejudices and anxieties that exist in the workplace occasionally. Even after your cancer treatment is finished, you might experience discrimination at work. Inform the human resources department of any potential employment discrimination problems you may be experiencing. If there is a union at your place of employment, its representatives might be useful resources for information on sickness and the workplace.

Keep a record of your interactions with office staff, including the names of the individuals you interacted with, the time and location of your conversations, and the details you learned. Additionally, it's a good idea to maintain copies of any written information about your work, including job performance reviews. If issues arise later, these can be very beneficial.

If you wish to complain about discrimination you can submit a complaint with the United States Equal Employment Opportunity Commission (EEOC) if you believe that you have experienced disability-based workplace discrimination. You have 180 days from the time you believe the discrimination occurred to take this action (although some states or local laws allow you to take up to 300 days).

CONCLUSION

A strategy for the detection and treatment of cancer is an essential part of any comprehensive cancer control strategy. Its primary objective is to either completely cure cancer patients or greatly extend their lives while ensuring a high quality of life. A diagnostic and treatment plan should never be created in a vacuum if it is to be effective. It must be connected to a program for early detection in order to identify patients when they are still treatable and more likely to be cured. Additionally, it needs to be combined with a palliative care program to provide patients with advanced cancers who are no longer candidates for treatment with enough comfort from their physical, emotional, and spiritual suffering. Additionally, programs must have an awareness-raising element to inform patients, family members, and community members about the variables that increase the risk of cancer and the importance of taking precautions to avoid getting it. When resources are scarce, diagnosis and treatment services should concentrate on all individuals presenting with cancers that can be cured, such as early-stage breast, cervical, and oral cancers. Acute lymphatic leukemia in children is another possibility; it has a good chance of being cured but cannot be caught early. Above all, services must be delivered in a sustainable and fair way. The program can be expanded to cover other diseases that can be cured as well as cancers for which treatment can significantly extend survival if more resources become available.